Essential Oil Recipes

THE COMPLETE GUIDE, HEALTH, HEALING, ANTI AGING, AND BEAUTY REFERENCE

OVER 700 ESSENTIAL OILS RECIPES INCLUSIVE.

(Essential oils recipes for beginners....aromatherapy book)

CARLA WHITES

Limit of Liability

The information in this book is solely for informational purposes, not as a medical instruction to replace the advice of your physician or as a replacement for any treatment prescribed by your physician. The author and publisher do not take responsibility for any possible consequences from any treatment, procedure, exercise, dietary modification, action or application of medication which results from reading or following the information contained in this book.

If you are ill or suspect that you have a medical problem, we strongly encourage you to consult your medical, health, or other competent professional before adopting any of the suggestions in this book or drawing inferences from it.

This book and the author's opinions are solely for informational and educational purposes. The author specifically disclaims all responsibility for any liability, loss, or risk, personal or otherwise which is incurred as a consequence, directly or indirectly, of the use and application of any of the contents of this book.

ISBN-13: 978-1544095974

ISBN-10: 154409597X

DEDICATION

To all who desire to live life to the fullest!

TABLE OF CONTENT

INTRODUCTION

This complete, concise, and simple guide to essential oils, their safety and their uses; was written to help you understand how essential oils are used, their uses therapeutically, and the facts about essential oils and so on.

The author of Aromatherapy: Soothing Remedies to Restore, Rejuvenate and Heal, Valerie Gennari Cooksley sees essential oils as very concentrated constituents of a plant that has cosmetic and medicinal properties. Essential oils are not oils in the real sense, since they don't have the fatty acids property that defines what we would accept as oil in actual sense.

Another keen perspective to essential oils definition was Stephanie Tourles. She believed essential oils were the soul and life core of a plant. Essential oils have high antifungal, antibacterial and antiviral properties; with these qualities, essential oils become a great and highly sought-after visitor in several homes. Some essential oils work very well when added to cleaning solutions prepared at home. Examples of essential Oils that are very used to clean are: Grape fruit, lemon, eucalyptus, tea tree, peppermint, rosemary and lavender.

The skin absorbs these oils well, because they are minuscule in molecular size. This makes them perfect additions to personal care recipes with the motive to make soft, nourish and heal the skin. Another good thing about essential oils is that over time they don't store up in the body, rather they heal, soften and nourish the body. We have it in record that inhaling some oils can help the brain extensively; example rosemary essential oil.

In this scientific study, two groups were tested and one of the groups inhaled no odor at all, and the other group inhaled either lavender or rosemary essential oil. The group that inhaled felt very much relaxed compared to those that did not inhale any essential oil.

There is a huge difference between an essential oil and fragrance oil. In fact if the word "perfume", "fragrance oil" or "fragrance" is written on the label of any beauty care bottle, you are right to believe the content would be synthetic.

NOTE: Even if it reads that is natural.

Essential oils are always very concentrated, because they are produced from great quantities of plant. For instance, you produce 1 lb. of essential oil from 4000 lbs. of Bulgarian roses. Some other plants take lesser lbs. of plant material to manufacture their essential oils; for instance, 1 lb. of Lavender essential oil is gotten from 100 lbs. of lavender plant.

Be very careful, you should never use most essential oils on your skin undiluted. Rather, the essential oils should be combined or diluted with carrier oils (also known as "real" oils), alcohols, butters, waxes or any diluting measure. Essential oils are very concentrated and can lead to unfortunate incidents and reactions on the skin, if used without diluting.

There are few oils that are widely accepted as danger free to use without diluting. Essential oils that are recognized generally and acknowledged as danger free to be used without diluting are: German chamomile, lavender, tea tree, rose geranium and sandal wood. This list is subjective, and essential oils should still be approached with caution.

Don't ever use oils on your children without diluting. A child has a thinner and very fragile skin compared to an adult, and children tend to react to essential oils potency. While administering essential oils to a child, divide the recommended essential oil recipe into two halves, and administer one portion.

CHAPTER ONE - ESSENTIAL FACTS OF ESSENTIAL OILS

Aromatherapy and Essential Oils

The use of essential oils in aromatherapy cannot be overemphasized. Essential oils have the capacity to help our emotions positively. Without using sprays or chemicals, essential oils can fragrance to the home.

Some of my greatest high points in the use of essential oils in aromatherapy include nebulizer diffusion, massage, burning oil as incense and heating the oil over a candle.

It is worthy of note to remember that essential oils should always be carefully handled. Essential oils that are not diluted can cause severe skin and health conditions if not handled in the right way; it is therefore important that you are adequately prepared before you begin to use essential oils.

Essential oils should not be applied directly to the skin unless you have diluted the essential oil within carrier oils. Examples of those carrier oils include olive oil, grape seed oil, hazelnut oil or almond oil. Carrier oils help to dilute essential oils so that you can apply to your skin without damaging the oil quality.

Essential Oils, what are they?

Is it possible to live a natural lifestyle, a world of smelling sweet and out of these world fragrances from natural sources? And also getting to receive the helps of aromatherapy! Yes it is definitely very possible and it is not farfetched. It is possible to have it.

Essential Oils are the oils gotten from plant sources. Examples of essential oils are neroli, peppermint and lemon which can be retrieved in 3 ways:

1. Distillation

2. Cold Press

NOTE: The first two are great ways to extract the oils

3. Solvent Extraction (the use of chemicals to retrieve essential oils)

Essential Safety Precaution

1. Avoid essential oil contact with your eyes.

2. All essential oils should be stored out of your child's reach.

3. Do not ingest essential oils, especially essential oils like eucalyptus and wintergreen.

NOTE: Some well diluted essential oils can be added to things like toothpaste with caution, but it is widely accepted that essential oils should not be taken internally.

4. There are many essential oils that are toxic to the skin and should be avoided through contact with the skin.

Be very cautious. The good news is that most of these toxic essential oils cannot be found in the store.

Essential Oils that works well for Personal Use

The essential oils listed below are some of the very available and least expensive essential oils around.

Lavender: Lavender essential oil works well for hair preparations, used for relaxation, great for all skin types and cleaning products.

Lemon: Lemon essential oil works well in cleaning preparations, lifting moods and sparingly in toners and products for oily skin.

Peppermint: Peppermint essential oil works well for oily/acneic skin remedies, good for lip balms, and cleaning products.

Rosemary: Rosemary essential oil work wells for oily/acneic skin remedies, is good for hair preparations, and cleaning products.

Tea tree: Tea tree essential oil works well for dandruff treatment, is great for healing, oily/acneic skin, and cleaning products.

Rose geranium: This essential oil is good for all skin types, making homemade moisturizers and creating perfumes.

Sweet orange: sweet orange essential oil works as very soothing spray for children's room and is good for all skin types.

Essential oils test

It is important to test for sensitivity before using an essential oil. It is the best thing to do before you use essential oil for skin care. To test:

Ingredients

1 drop of essential oil

1/2 teaspoon jojoba, olive oil or sweet almond (carrier oils).

Instructions:

1. Combine the essential oil with the carrier oil together

2. Rub the mixture on the inside part of your upper side of your arm and wait a couple of hours.

3. If you are sensitive to the essential oil, an itching or redness will develop.

CHAPTER TWO-BENEFITS OF ESSENTIAL OILS

Essential Oils were once known as aromatic oils, they have been around for many centuries, and several world civilizations and cultures used them. Many cultures and civilizations had different use for essential oils. To some It was for the purpose of healing, to others it was mainly religious, and to some others it was both.

We cannot ascertain the exact time that the popularity of essential oils as efficient healing agents began. What's important is that essential oils knowledge eventually found its way into many cultures and every part of the globe.

In Lascaux, a small region of Dordogne in France, the first evidences that suggests that early humans knew about plants' healing properties is evident from the Paleolithic cave paintings which suggest the regular use of medical plants on daily basis. These paleolithic cave paintings were carbon-dated to be around 18,000 Before Common Era.

For thousands of years, essential oils have been used for various purposes in different civilizations and cultures.

Essential oils have been used for aromatherapy, health and for purposes of medicine, household cleaning products, natural medicine treatments and personal beauty care.

Essential oils may have particles and these particles come from extracting and distilling the different parts of the plants, which include their flowers, leaves, roots, barks, peels and resins. Thousands of years ago, Egyptian and the

Jews produced essential oils by soaking the plants in oil and then they filter it using a linen bag.

There are several benefits gotten from essential oils, some of the benefits comes from their antimicrobial, anti-inflammatory and antioxidant properties. These essential oils have notoriety as healing oils because they act as natural medicine without side effects.

Essential Oil Uses for the Home and Cleaning

All purpose cleaner

1. Combine 3 drops of tea tree oil and another 3 drops of lemon oil together.

2. Mix into a few ounces of water that is warm.

2. To disinfect naturally, spray essential oil mixture on countertops.

Lean Cleats, Jerseys and Sports gear

1. Toss 2 drops of lemon oil and 2 drops of tea tree oil into 1 qt of warm water.

2. Toss in 4 tbsps of baking soda into the tea tree/lemon mixture.

3. Combine to mix

4. Use mixture to lean cleats, jerseys and sports gear.

For Repelling Mosquitoes

1. Mix a drop of citronella oil, another drop of lemongrass oil and one drop of eucalyptus.

2. Combine with 1 tsp of coconut oil.

3. Rub on your skin to repel mosquitoes naturally.

1. Spray cinnamon oil into the air and you have a clean and fresh air.

NOTE: one of the benefits of cinnamon essential oil is that it has antimicrobial properties.

Keeping Your Washing Machine Fresh

1. Mix in approx. 10 to 20 drops of essential oil mixture of your choice.

2. Drizzle into washing machine per wash.

Peppermint Patties

1. Combine coconut oil, peppermint oil, raw honey and dark chocolate.

2. Mix together until well incorporated.

Sunscreen

To make a sunscreen that is toxic free;

1. Combine zinc oxide, coconut oil, shea butter, lavender oil and helichrysum oil together.

2. Store mixture in a bottle that can be squeezed.

Vacuum Cleaner

1. In your dust container or vacuum bag,

2. Mix in 5 to 10 drops of your favorite essential oil.

Removing Shower Curtain Scum

1. Get a 16 oz. spray bottle,

2. Add 4 drops of tea tree oil and 4 drops of eucalyptus oil with warm water.

3. Spray essential oil mixture into your shower to kill mold.

Sweet Smelling Home

1. Combine 1-2 drops each of rosemary oil, clove oil, and orange oil.

2. Spray into the air and it will give your home that natural fragrance.

Burnt Pan Cleaning

1. Combine 3 drops of lemon oil with boiling water.

2. Apply to pans and pots to remove burnt food.

Carpet Cleaner

1. Combine Borax and 20 drops of tea tree oil into a bowl,

2. Use to clean your carpet.

Lavender Cake

1. Combine lavender oil, raw honey, coconut flour and organic eggs.

2. Mix well until batter thickens consistently.

3. Bake in an oven at 350oF.

Pesticide

1. Combine few drops of clove oil and orange oil together.

2. Spray mixture on pests. It kills immediately.

To Remove Mold

1. Diffuse tea tree oil into the air.

2. The diffused oil will kill pathogens and mold in the air.

Christmas Scent

1. Combine one drop of sandalwood oil and a drop of pine oil with another drop of cedarwood oil.

2. On a log, toss essential oil mixture.

NOTE: Toss oil onto log approx. 30 minutes before you burn the log.

For Enlightenment Spiritually

1. Get frankincense oil,

2. When you pray, read or meditate, spray frankincense into the air to increase spiritual awareness.

To Reduce Anxiety

1. Get lavender oil,

2. Spray the oil around your house to calm your nerves and reduce tension and stress feelings.

To Freshen Trash Can

1. Combine 2 drops of tea tree oil and 2 drops of lemon oil.

2. Mix to combine.

3. Soak cotton ball into the essential oil mixture and place at the bottom of a trash can to reduce foul odor and to detoxify.

Bathtub Scrub

1. Combine 1/2 cup of vinegar and 1/2 cup of baking soda with 5 drops of lime oil or bergamot oil as a substitute.

2. Mix well.

3. Apply to scrub bathtub or sink.

To Wash Farm Produce

1. In a clean bowl of water, toss in 2 drops of lemon oil,

2. Mix thoroughly to combine.

3. Use bowl of water mixture to wash vegetables and fruits.

To Eliminate Kitchen Smell

1. Combine 3 drops of cinnamon oil and 3 drops of clove oil with 3 drops of citrus oil.

2. Mix well to combine.

3. To get rid of cooking odors, toss mixture into a simmering pan of water.

For A Purified Refrigerator

1. Add 3-5 drops of lime, grapefruit or bergamot essential oil to a bowl of water.

2. Combine essential oil well

3. Use water mixture to clean freezer or fridge to freshen it up.

Bathroom Freshener

1. Get lemon/lime essential oil,

2. Soak cotton ball into essential oil mixture.

3. Place essential oil soaked cotton ball behind the toilet. Your bathroom will be freshened

Mint Tea

1. Get 1 to 2 drops of peppermint oil.

2. Add peppermint essential oil into your favorite tea.

To Detoxify The Air

1. Combine few drops of eucalyptus and few drops of peppermint oil.

2. Mix well to combine.

3. Toss essential oil mixture into 1 gallon of paint.

4. Use to dispel fumes.

To Get Rid Of Smoke

1. Combine 4 drops of tea tree oil and 4 drops of rosemary oil with 4 drops of eucalyptus oil into a spray bottle.

2. Mix well.

3. Spray into the air to eliminate cigarette smoke.

Get Rid Of Shoe Smell

1. Combine few drops of lemon oil and few drops of tea tree oil together.

2. Mix very well.

3. Toss few drops to the shoes to get rid of foul odors from shoes.

Gift For Baby Shower

1. Add the right amount of lavender essential oil to a diffuser.

2. Spray to calm baby and mother.

Gift For Bridal Shower

1. Combined 20 drops of sandalwood oil, 4 drops of cocoa, rose oil and vanilla oil to unscented lotion.

2. This serves as great gift for a bridal shower, it creates an atmosphere of love.

Flavored Lemon Water

1. Get a bowl of water,

2. Measure in 2 to 3 drops of lemon oil into it.

Drug Cabinet

1. For a handy first aid box or drug cabinet,

2. Store lavender, peppermint, lemon, tea tree, frankincense and oregano essential oils in it.

Sparkling Dishes

1. In a dishwasher, add 3 to 4 drops of lemon oil

NOTE: Add the lemon oil essential oil before you wash.

You can be sure of a spot free sparkling wash.

Essential Oil Uses Relaxation and Spa

To Improve Your Sleep

1. Get lavender oil,

2. Drizzle 3 to 4 drops of lavender oil on your pillow.

3. It will help eliminate insomnia and help you sleep well.

Homemade Lip Balm

To heal chapped lips,

1. Mix beeswax oil, with coconut oil and lavender oil, together.

2. Mix well.

3. Apply to affected body part for healing.

Body Butter Lotion

1. Combine coconut oil, magnesium oil and Shea butter and your favorite oils for moisturizing, together.

2. Mix well.

3. Apply to the body as a moisturizing body lotion.

To Relieve Tension

1. Get lavender essential oil,

2. Add 1 drop of lavender oil to your hands.

3. Rub your hands together, so that essential oil will spread consistently across your palm.

4. Cup your lavender coated hands to your nostrils and allow the scent permeate you and relieve you of anxiety.

For Instant Relaxation

1. Combine 2 to 4 drops of lavender oil, 2 to 4 drops of chamomile oil and 2 to 4 drops of peppermint oil.

2. Mix well

3. Apply mixtures to your temple. You will have a cool feel and you will become immediately relaxed on application.

Massage Therapy

1. Combine 3 to 4 drops of lavender oil or cedarwood oil with any lotion that is unscented.

2. Mix well.

3. Apply during massage to relax.

Detox Bath

1. Combine Epsom salts, lavender oil and sea salt together.

2. Mix well.

3. Add mixtures to warm bath.

Your body will be rejuvenated and cleansed.

To Calm A Child That Is Upset

1. Combine few drops of lavender oil and few drops of chamomile oil together.

2. Mix well.

3. Apply mixture to your child's stuffed animal to sooth and calm them.

Sauna Therapy

1. In a sauna, add 2 drops of any essential oil of your choice into 2 cups of water.

2. Mix to combine well.

Foot Bath

1. Combine 2 to 3 drops eucalyptus oil or lemon oil with warm water.

2. Mix thoroughly.

3. Apply to your feet to soothe.

Yoga And Pilates

1. Inhale sandalwood oil or lavender oil before yoga class;

2. Combine citrus oil and clove oil together.

3. Use citrus mixture to clean the yoga mats before meditation. These helps you relax while meditating or during yoga.

Improve Depression

1. To eliminate mood swings, add rose oil to your inhalations, baths, and diffusers to help boost your mood.

Mint Chocolate Cocoa

1. Make a hot cup of cocoa,

2. Toss in 2 to 3 drops of peppermint oil and mix.

Essential Oil Uses for Skin and Beauty

To Reduce Cellulite

1. Combine 2 tsps of coconut oil with 5 drops of grapefruit oil.

2. Massage oil mixture into dimpled areas.

Face Wash For Acne

1. Combine raw honey and tea tree oil together.

2. Apply to your face to rid your face of acne.

3. Rinse your face off with water.

Natural Perfume

1. Apply 1 to 2 drops of jasmine oil to your wrist. It acts as a fresh natural fragrance.

2. Clove oil and cypress oil can be used as a substitute for men's cologne.

3. Vanilla and lavender oils are perfect for most women.

To Freshen Breath

1. Add 1 drop of peppermint oil.

2. Apply to freshen your breathe naturally.

Domestic Deodorant

1. Mix beeswax and coconut oil together,

2. Mix with your favorite oils like tea tree essential oil and lavender essential oil for women, and clove oil or cedarwood oil for men

Shampoo Made At Home

1. Combine rosemary oil, lavender oil, coconut milk and aloe vera gel.

2. Apply to hair the same way you would a regular shampoo.

Salt Or Sugar Scrub

1. Combine 2 to 3 drops of any essential oil and almond oil,

2. Add to sugar or rock salt.

To Correct Itchy Scalp

1. Get a regular shampoo,

2. Toss in few drops of lavender oil, basil oil or cedarwood oil into the shampoo.

3. Apply on scalp to eliminate itching.

Toothpaste Made At Home

1. Mix baking soda, sea salt and coconut oil.

2. Mix with xylitol and peppermint oil.

This makes a great remineralizing toothpaste for a great wash.

To Thicken Hair

1. Get a regular shampoo,

2. Add rosemary oil to it.

3. Apply on hair to make your hair become thick naturally and increase its volume.

To Reduce Wrinkles

1. Combine 3 to 5 drops of sandalwood oil, lavender oil, geranium oil and frankincense oil together.

2. Mix with a lotion that is unscented.

3. Rub on face; avoid application to the eyes.

To Strengthen Nails

1. Combine 10 drops of myrrh oil, frankincense oil and lemon oil together,

2. Mix into 2 tbsps of vitamin E oil,

3. Apply to cuticles.

To Whiten Your Teeth

1. Mix coconut oil, fresh strawberries, and lemon oil together.

2. Apply on your teeth.

3. Rinse your teeth off after 2 minutes.

To Control Stretch Marks

1. Combine 5 drops of myrrh oil, 5 drops of frankincense oil and 5 drops of grapefruit oil together.

2. Mix mixture with coconut oil.

3. Rub on stretch marks

To Cure Dandruff

1. Combine 5 drops of rosemary oil and 5 drops of lavender oil together.

2. Mix with 3 tbsps of unscented oil.

3. Apply by massaging into your scalp.

4. Shampoo it out after 10 minutes.

Facial Scrub

1. Combine 1/4 cup cornmeal, 1/4 cup yogurt together,

2. Add mixture to 5 drops of patchouli oil, lavender oil and grapefruit oil.

3. Rub on the face, leave for a while, then rinse off.

Deep Hair Conditioner

1. Combine 5 drops of sandalwood oil and 5 drops of lavender with 15 drops of rosewood oil.

2. Mix into an unscented oil.

3. Transfer mixture into a resealable plastic bag and dip into warm water to warm mixture up and wrap for about 20 minutes.

4. Apply as you would a regular shampoo

Natural Skin Toner

1. Combine 2 drops of lavender oil, 2 drops of frankincense oil, and 2 drops of geranium oil.

2. Mix lavender/geranium essential oil mixture with 8 oz. of water.

3. Apply to the skin.

Reduce Age Spots

1. Apply few drops of frankincense oil to your skin directly.

2. Do this three times a day to improve and gradually correct age spots and sun spots.

For Dry Cracked Feet Healing

1. Combine 3 drops of lavender oil to 2 tbsps of coconut oil.

2. Rub on dry cracked feet before you go to bed.

3. After application, put some socks on.

For Oily Hair

1. Combine 10 drops of lime oil, ylang ylang oil and rosemary oil.

2. Combine with 2 oz. of unscented oil (about 1/4 cup).

3. Apply to scalp 2 to 3 times in a week.

4. Wash out after a while.

To Relieve Nausea

1. To eliminate nausea, inhale peppermint oil through your nostrils.

2. You can also rub peppermint oil on your upper chest and neck,

3. Lavender and Ginger oils can also be a good substitute for peppermint oil.

Essential Oil Natural Medicine and Remedies

Headache Relief For Migraine

1. Come 3-4 drops of peppermint oil and 3-4 drops of lavender oil.

2. Rub on your temple to eliminate migraines and headaches.

To Fix Broken Bones

1. Combine few drops of fir oil, helichrysum oil and cypress oil.

2. Apply to support broken bone recovery.

Reduce Sinusitis or Cough

1. Combine 5-7 drops of eucalyptus oil into a few ounces of very hot water or into a diffuser.

2. Draw in through your nose, to clear the nasal passage.

To Heal Burns

1. Combine aloe vera with lavender essential oil.

2. Apply to burns.

To Improve Your Digestion

1. Mix peppermint oil, ginger oil and fennel oil.

2. Take to help improve your digestion and to heal leaky gut.

To Soothe Bug Bites

1. Get few drops of lavender essential oil,

2. Apply to stings and bug bites.

Asthma And Bronchitis Remedy

1. Mix few drops of peppermint oil, eucalyptus oil and coconut oil.

2. Rub on the neck and upper chest.

Improve Concentration

1. To increase and improve your concentration during your daily activities, inhale bergamot essential oil.

2. Grapefruit oil or peppermint oil are great replacements also.

To Treat Bruises

1. Combine 5 drops of frankincense and 5 drops of lavender.

2. Mix into 4 oz. of water (1/2 cup) and soak.

3. Apply to bruises.

To Soak Sore Feet

1. Combine 1 tbsp of Epsom salt and 10 drops of peppermint together.

2. Mix into foot bath with warm water.

3. Apply by washing feet.

To Relieve PMS

1. Combine 2 drops of basil oil, 2 drops of sage oil and 2 drops of rosemary.

2. Rosemary/basil oil mixture should be applied to a warm and moist towel.

3. The towel should then be applied to the abdomen.

To Reduce Teeth Grinding

1. Get 1-3 drops of lavender essential oil,

2. Apply by rubbing it into the back of your ears and massaging it into the sole of your feet, before go to bed.

Psoriasis And Eczema Cream

1. Combine Shea butter and few drops of lavender essential oil.

2. Apply to psoriasis and eczema affected skin area.

Relieve Hangover Symptoms

1. Combine 6 drops of cedarwood oil, 6 drops of juniper berry oil, 6 drops of grapefruit oil, 6 drops of rosemary oil, 6 drops of lavender oil and 6 drops of lemon oil.

2. Mix into a warm water bath.

To Improve Circulation

1. Toss 8 to 10 drops of grapefruit oil into a warm bath water.

2. Wash your body with the warm water treatment.

To Balance Blood Sugar And Control Food Cravings

1. Combine cinnamon oil and peppermint oil,

2. Draw mixture in through the nose to decrease appetite and balance blood sugar.

To Reduce Fever

1. Mix 1 to 3 drops of peppermint oil, 1 to 3 drops of eucalyptus oil and 1 to 3 drops of lavender oil.

2. Toss mix into a cool cloth and apply on the body, use cloth as a sponge.

To Energize Your Workout

1. Before working out inhale peppermint essential oil.

2. Inhale also to decrease tiredness.

To Relieve Motion Sickness

1. Combine few drops of lavender oil, few drops of peppermint oil and few drops of ginger oil.

2. Apply to relieve motion sickness.

To Treat Ringworm

1. Mix 3 drops of coconut oil and 3 drops of tea tree oil.

2. Apply by massaging into the affected areas.

3. Apply 2 times a day.

For Arthritis Relief

1. Combine 2 drops of cypress oil, 2 drops of wintergreen oil and 2 drops of lemon grass oil.

2. Mix into unscented lotion.

3. Apply by massaging into affected areas.

To Cure Head Lice

1. Combine 3 drops of lavender oil, 3 drops of thyme oil and 3 drops of eucalyptus oil.

2. Mix into an oil that is unscented.

3. Apply and cover your head with a shower cap.

4. Leave on the scalp for approx. 30 minutes.

5. Wash scalp out.

To Soothe A Sunburn

1. Mix few drops of chamomile oil and few drops of lavender oil.

2. Mix with 1 tbsp of coconut oil.

3. Use a cotton ball to apply to affected skin area.

It reduces the pain and the swelling.

For Blistered Skin Healing

1. Combine 2 drops of unscented oil and 2 drops of tea tree oil.

2. Apply to the affected area.

3. Apply five different times daily.

To Treat Poison Ivy Or Poison Oak

1. Combine 3 drops of peppermint essential oil and few drops of an unscented oil;

2. Apply to the area affected.

Immune System Boost

1. Combine 1 drop of oregano and 4 drops of any carrier oil.

2. Apply by rubbing on the sole of your feet before you fly in an airplane.

To Lose Weight

1. Mix few drops of ginger oil, few drops of grapefruit oil and few drops of cinnamon oil.

2. Ingest as a food supplement thrice per day to help metabolism.

Rub For Achy Muscle

1. Combine few drops of wintergreen oil, few drops of eucalyptus oil and few drips of cypress oil.

2. Mix into an unscented lotion.

3. Apply to affected areas.

Improving Allergies

1. Mix few drops of lavender oil and few drops of frankincense oil.

2. Apply mixture to your palms and rub.

3. Inhale through your nose for itchy throat and itchy eyes relief.

Reducing Pregnancy-Caused Morning Sickness

1. Apply 2 to 3 drops of lemon oil, 2 to 3 drops of wild orange oil, or 2 to 3 drops of ginger oil to a handkerchief.

2. Inhale through the nose.

Get Rid Of Cold Fast

1. Combine 3 drops of frankincense oil and 3 drops of oregano oil.

2. Take 3 drops 3 times per day for 1 week.

To Reduce Neck And Back Pain

1. Mix few drops of cypress oil, few drops of peppermint oil and few drops of ginger oil.

2. Mix with cayenne pepper and coconut oil.

3. Apply by rubbing on affected areas.

Quality of an Essential Oil

The most important thing to note about an essential is its quality. Not every essential oil was equally created. Often times, most of them are actually useless to your health and most times synthetic. Therefore it becomes very important and crucial to ascertain the authenticity of an essential oil, when buying it. Make sure an essential oil has been certified as pure therapeutic grade, before buying.

CHAPTER THREE – THE AROMATIC BLENDING OF ESSENTIAL OILS

Aromatic blending is a combination of the depth of science and the creativity of art. A blend could be created primarily for its aroma; therapeutic benefits can still be gotten from such blends, notwithstanding. However, the focus of the blend is not on the therapeutic benefits but on the final aroma that would be gotten.

It is important to adhere to outlined safety precautions during aromatic blending and any other type of blending.

For example, you have to be very careful when handling Bergamot because of its phototoxic properties. You also need to avoid the use of oils that are hazardous, and oils that have contraindications for the conditions you have.

It takes several years to master the science and art of perfumery blending. In aromatherapy blending, only natural ingredients are used compared to perfumery blending and the likes. Ingredients such as, essential oils,

CO2s, absolutes, grain alcohol, herbs, carrier oils and water are used. Since aromatherapy blending relies completely on the use of natural and unsynthesized chemicals; aromatherapy blending would not replicate your favorite commercial fragrances perfectly.

Commonly Available Essential Oils Chart

Top Notes

Basil

Anise

Bergamot

Bay Laurel

Citronella

Bergamot Mint

Galbanum

Eucalyptus

Lavender

Grapefruit

Lemon

Lavendin

Lime

Lemongrass

Peppermint

Orange

Spearmint

Petitgrain

Tangerine

Tagetes

Middle Notes

Bois-de-rose

Bay

Carrot Seed

Cajeput

Chamomile, Roman

Chamomile, German

Clary Sage

Cinnamon

Cypress

Clove Bud

Elemi

Dill

Fir Needle

Fennel

Hyssop

Geranium

Juniper Berry

Jasmine

Marjoram

Linden Blossom

Nutmeg

Neroli

Parsley

Palmarosa

Pine, Scotch

Pepper, Black

Rose Geranium

Rose

Rosewood

Rosemary

Tea Tree, Common

Spruce

Thyme

Tea Tree, NZ (Manuka)

Yarrow

Tobacco

Ylang Ylang

Base Notes

Angelica Root

Beeswax

Balsam, Peru

Cedarwood, Atlas

Benzoin

Frankincense

Cedarwood, Virginian

Ginger

Myrrh

Helichrysum (Immortelle)

Olibanum

Oakmoss

Sandalwood

Patchouli

Vetiver

Vanilla

Essential Oils Home-Made Perfume

Making your own perfume isn't as difficult as it sounds.
For a long time I wore store bought perfumes, enjoying
the beautiful floral scents, having no doubts whatsoever
about the perfumes I used.

Not long ago I started to look into the chemicals used in
producing my beauty and skin care products. To my
shock, I found hidden chemicals in many of beauty and
skin care staples which includes my perfume.

While many body sprays, deodorants, antiperspirants and
perfumes claims being natural with citrus, floral and exotic

fragrances - they are very much synthetic. And more so manufacturers are not obliged to disclose ingredients (such as fragrances and synthetic chemicals), because these ingredients are regarded as production trade secrets.

In some laboratory tests that the Campaign for Safe Cosmetics commissioned, the Environmental Working Group (EWG) discovered

1. Thirty eight secret chemicals in Seventeen name brand fragrances.

These fragrances include;

2. Britney Spears Curious - Seventeen chemicals {not listed},

3. Coco Chanel - Eighteen chemicals {not listed}, and

4. Giorgio Armani Acqua Di Gio - Seventeen chemicals {not listed}.

Many of these name brand fragrances contain secret chemicals that are associated with allergic reactions and endocrine disruption. Secondly most of these chemicals didn't undergo any assessment to check for safety.

This discovery helped me decide to stop buying name brand fragrances and start making my own perfumes.

The Perfume Basics

Making your own perfume is not a herculean task as it may seem. It takes few essential oils and few base ingredients to make that fragrant blend you have always wanted.

The fragrance of a perfume has three classifications. The fragrance is classified into what is called "notes".

There are three notes, such as;

1. The Top Note:

This is the first impression you get from the perfume, it is always light and it evaporates very quickly.

Examples are lemon, grapefruit, orange, lime, citronella, tangerine, bergamot, lavender, eucalyptus, peppermint, lemongrass and spearmint.

2. The Middle Note

This is the major fragrance of the perfume, it is soft, sweet and calm, and it comes out few minutes after the top notes.

Examples are chamomile, clove, cinnamon, cypress, geranium, fennel, jasmine, marjoram, juniper, neroli, pine, nutmeg, fir, rosemary, rose, tea tree, spruce, ylang ylang and thyme.

3. The Base Note

This is the rich part and deep fragrance of the perfume, and most times a musk fragrance.

Examples are cedarwood, ginger, frankincense, helichrysum, patchouli, myrrh, sandalwood, vetiver and vanilla.

Types of Aromas

You can also classify essential oils as aromas or scents

1. Floral: Rose, lavender, geranium, and jasmine.

2. Earthy: Patchouli and vetiver.

3. Woodsy: Pine and cedar.

4. Minty: Peppermint.

5. Herbaceous: Basil and rosemary.

6. Spicy: Nutmeg, clove and cinnamon.

7. Camphorous: Eucalyptus.

8. Citrus: Lemon and orange.

9. Oriental: Ginger

Producing your own Perfume

Making your own perfumes is simple based on blending your favorite aromas and mixing with a carrier oil. For example floral/spicy or citrus/exotic. Below are few blend examples that you can work around.

Grapefruit/Ylang Ylang (Energizing Blend)

1. Combine 7 drops of grapefruit and 4 drops of Ylang Ylang.

2. Mix into a 5ml roller bottle,

3. Add in fractionated coconut oil or sweet almond oil

Fractioned coconut oil is odorless and doesn't become solid when cold.

Lavender/Vetiver/Lemon (Woodsy Blend)

1. Combine 5 drops of lavender, 3 drops of vetiver and 4 drops of lemon.

2. Mix into a 5ml roller bottle,

3. Add in fractionated coconut oil or sweet almond oil

Fractioned coconut oil is odorless and doesn't become solid when cold.

Jasmine/Lime (Floral Blend)

1. Combine 7 drops of Jasmine and 4 drops of lime.

2. Mix into a 5ml roller bottle,

3. Add in fractionated coconut oil or sweet almond oil

Fractioned coconut oil is odorless and doesn't become solid when cold.

Lavender/Copaiba/Lime (Sexy Musk Blend)

1. Combine 5 drops of lavender, 3 drops of copaiba and 4 drops of lime.

2. Mix into a 5ml roller bottle,

3. Add in fractionated coconut oil or sweet almond oil

Fractioned coconut oil is odorless and doesn't become solid when cold.

CHAPTER FOUR- ESSENTIAL OILS FOR BEAUTY

Whipped Shea Butter

Recipe works perfectly for your skin. This recipe is light, creamy and soft and contains all the nourishment that Shea butter and the other essential oil added in the ingredient has. The consistency of Whipped Shea Butter is similar to that of whipped cream. It is a bit tricky and time consuming to make, but the results are well worth it.

Ingredients

Makes: approx. four (4 oz.) jars of whipped Shea butter

8 net wt. oz. Shea Butter

1/2 teaspoon Vitamin E Oil (preferably T-50 or T-80)

1 tablespoon Jojoba

1/16 teaspoon Pearlescent Mica Powder for Color (if desired)

1/4 teaspoon Essential Oil

Instructions

1. Get an all-temperature jumbo sized mixing bowl,

NOTE: Mixing bowl should be able to withstand hot/cold temperatures.

Your freezer should be able to accommodate the size of the bowl.

2. Boil water in the lower portion of a double boiler.

3. Lower heat to medium high.

4. In the top portion of the double boiler, toss in Shea butter and leave until its melted, stirring frequently.

5 Adjust the temperature of the stove until the Shea butter is at 175°F, using a candy thermometer. Keep heating for 20 minutes at 175°F.

NOTE: Heating higher than 175°F would damage some Shea butter constituents that are nutritive. Be watchful as you heat the

Shea butter, Shea butter is flammable.

6. Quickly and carefully transfer heated Shea butter into the jumbo sized mixing bowl.

7. Toss in vitamin E oil and jojoba very quickly.

8. Using a mixer, whisk Shea butter until well mixed for about 5 to 10 minutes.

9. Remove mixing bowl from the freezer, the Shea butter at this time would still be in a liquid stage, though a film of Shea butter that is solid may have formed.

10. Mix Shea butter for 5 to 10 minutes.

NOTE: Repeat the process of mixing Shea butter and returning to the freezer severally. Keep repeating until a firm and consistent Shea butter is gotten. It should look like frosting or whipped cream. It takes a lot of practice to get this things right. Quick freezing the Shea butter for a short while per interval is very important as this will help enhance, expedite and maintain the whipped cream texture of the whipped butter. It is also very important that you don't over freeze the whipped Shea butter, and don't mix for too long either, to prevent whipped Shea butter from becoming gritty.

11. Toss in the essential oils of your choice, once Shea butter has reached frosting or whipped cream consistency.

NOTE: Adhere to all essential oil safety precautions when using any essential oil or blend.

12. Evenly distribute essential oils into whipped Shea butter by mixing well for several minutes.

13. For color, toss in the pearlescent mica powder and combine thoroughly.

14. Scoop into 4 oz. labeled containers; write the date of production on the label.

15. Store in a cool dry place, ensure clean hands when using and don't use for more than a month.

Cocoa Butter Stretch Mark Recipes

Nourishing and moisturizing the skin around the thighs and abdomen during pregnancy can reduce and probably completely eliminate the risks of having stretch marks during pregnancy. When the skin is adequately moisturized helps to maintain skin elasticity and prevent stretch marks when loosing significant amounts of weight.

The beauty of the recipe below is that they can be made without the addition of essential oil, as there are concerns as to whether a pregnant woman can be exposed to essential oils.

Cocoa butter comes with a sweet natural aroma, but you may have to consider the deodorized cocoa butter variant if the cocoa butter natural aroma conflicts with the essential oils choice you made.

Ingredients

3 net weight oz. Cocoa Butter

4 drops Neroli Essential Oil (if desired)

1 oz.fl., Avocado Oil (or any other carrier oil of choice)

4 oz. jar with a good cover.

Instructions

1. Melt cocoa butter gently in a double boiler.

2. Toss in avocado oil, stirring continuously.

3. Pour the essential oils mixture you are using carefully into a bowl, set aside to cool for a while.

NOTE: Essential oil evaporates easily when exposed to hot temperatures, so it's important to allow it cool for a while.

4. Add essential oils mixture into cocoa butter mixture and stir.

5. Pour mixture into the jar carefully and set aside to cool.

NOTE: The firmness or softness of your mixture is dependent on the room temperature, if the recipe turns out too soft, use lesser oil. If it turns out to firm, add more oil.

This blend can be used with essential oils famed to be helpful with stretch marks or any essential oil that you like.

It is worthy of note that you use only oils that are beneficial and safe for the skin.

6. Apply to your abdomen and upper thighs 2 times per day.

NOTE: Don't apply around the genital area. Stop using if you discover any sensitivity.

Liquid Shower Gel Recipe

Ingredients

70 drops of lavender (or any favorite essential oils of your choice)

7 oz. fl., Shower Gel Base, unscented

8 ounce bottle

Instructions

1. In a mixing bowl, toss in the shower gel base.

2. Blend in lavender oil or any other essential oil you are using.

3. Combine thoroughly.

4. Pour shower gel mixture into an 8 ounce bottle, using a funnel.

NOTE: Adhere to all essential oil safety precautions when using any essential oil or blend. Always do a skin patch test for essential oils before usage, make sure the essential oils you are using are gentle to the skin.

5. Use as you would a regular shower gel.

Shoe Deodorizer Recipe

Ingredients

4 tbsps baking soda

5-6 drops Lavender Essential Oil

4 tbsps cornstarch (preferably Non-GMO)

Instructions

1. Get a mixing bowl,

2. Combine baking soda and cornstarch together in the bowl.

3. Stir in lavender oil gradually until well incorporated.

4. Pour mixture in a well covered container and store in a cool dry place.

NOTE: You can use powder sifters containers.

5. Apply by sprinkling into shoes several hours before wearing the shoes, evening or overnight is a good time. Before putting shoes on, flip shoes over to get rid of contents of the shoes.

NOTE: Be careful when turning shoes over, to prevent the powder from harming the fragile shoe surfaces. You can add 4 more tbsps of baking soda if cornstarch can't be gotten.

Easy to make Aromatherapy Shampoo Recipe

Ingredients

7 fluid ounces Unscented Shampoo Base

40 drops Lavender essential Oil

1 tbsp Jojoba {if desired} (gives the hair added hydration)

5 drops Ylang Ylang essential Oil

10 drops Rosemary essential Oil

Instructions

1. Get a mixing bowl,

2. Toss in the unscented shampoo base into the bowl,

3. Blend in lavender, jojoba, ylang ylang and rosemary essential oils.

4. Combine thoroughly until essential oils are well incorporated.

5. Pour shampoo into an 8 ounce bottle, using a funnel.

NOTE: Adhere to all essential oil safety precautions when using any essential oil or blend. Always do a skin patch test for essential oils before usage, make sure the essential oils you are using are gentle to the skin.

6. Apply as you would a regular shampoo.

Scented Hair Aromatherapy Recipe

This recipe gives a lovely fragrance to your hair.

Ingredient

1 drop of Lavender/Rosemary/Sandalwood

Instructions

1. Choose any one of the essential oils listed in the ingredient list.

2. Apply 1 drop to the bristles of a hair brush.

3. Use hair brush to brush your hair thoroughly.

Natural Solid Perfume Recipe

Ingredients

Makes: Approx 1 oz. of solid perfume.

1/8 oz. Floral Wax/Beeswax

7 drops Essential Oil

1/2 oz. Jojoba

Instructions

1. Measure in floral wax or beeswax with jojoba into a double boiler.

2. Melt the wax mixture until completely melted.

3. Remove wax mixture from heat and set aside to cool.

NOTE: Mixture shouldn't be allowed to solidify

4. Toss in your favorite essential oil or essential oil blends.

5. Stir thoroughly to incorporate essential oil into the wax mixture.

6. Pour whole mixture into a suitable container.

NOTE: Do not handle containers while it is hot, allow container to cool completely before handling.

7. Apply as you would a regular perfume.

NOTE: If you added any phototoxic essential oils, do not apply to areas that would be exposed to sunlight directly.

8. Store in a cool, dry place. Recipe should not be used beyond 1 to 2 months.

NOTE: Adhere to all essential oil safety precautions when using any essential oil or blend. Always do a skin patch test for essential oils before usage, make sure the essential oils you are using are gentle to the skin.

Easy Natural Perfume Recipe

Ingredients

9 drops Sandalwood

1 tbsp Jojoba

3 drops Jasmine/Rose/Neroli (anyone that suits you)

Instructions

1. Get a dark colored container,

2. Blend sandalwood, jojoba and anyone of Jasmine, rose or neroli together. Blend well.

3. Dab to your pulse points as you would a regular perfume.

NOTE: Adhere to all essential oil safety precautions when using any essential oil or blend. Always do a skin patch test for essential oils before usage, make sure the essential oils you are using are gentle to the skin.

Essential oils Mouthwash Recipe

Ingredients

6 oz. fl., Water

4 drops Peppermint/spearmint Essential Oil

1-2 oz.fl., Vodka

3 drops Myrrh

8 ounce bottle

Instructions

1. In a bottle, mix water and vodka together.

2. Add in the essential oils,

3. Cover well, and then shake very well.

NOTE: Essential oils do not mix well in water based solutions. Therefore it is necessary to shake well before each use.

4. Apply as you would any regular mouthwash.

TIP: Vodka helps in killing germs and also helps to keep the essential oils emulsified.

Men's Cologne Recipe

This is natural, cool and very manly cologne for a man.

Ingredients

2.5 fluid ounces High Proof Vodka or Perfumer's Alcohol

15 drops Bergamot or Mandarin

1 fluid ounces Distilled Water

15 drops Patchouli

4 ounces glass bottle (with a sprayer top)

5 drops Oakmoss Absolute or 2-3 drops Vetiver

1-2 drops of Neroli (If desired)

3 drops Black Pepper or Ginger

5 drops Bay Laurel

Instructions

1. In a clean and sterilized glass bottle, mix water and alcohol.

2. Add in the essential oils and shake thoroughly.

3. Set aside for several days. Shake bottle vigorously twice a day even while cologne is set aside.

TIP: The setting aside helps the oil to blend well and mellow out before usage for the first time.

NOTE: Adhere to all essential oil safety precautions when using any essential oil or blend. Always do a skin patch test for essential oils before usage, make sure the essential oils you are using are gentle to the skin.

4. Shake well before you and apply as you would a regular cologne.

NOTE: Always shake well before each use to avoid essential oils concentration on your skin.

Natural Aromatherapy Hair Conditioner Recipe

This recipe is very easy to make.

Ingredients

Makes: 1 application

1-3 drops Rosemary Essential Oil

1 tbsp Jojoba

Instructions

1. In a tiny condiment bowl, combine rosemary essential oil and jojoba essential oil together.

2. Pour into a clean and sterile glass bottle.

NOTE: The ingredients can be increased to make a larger quantity.

3. Use hair conditioner by wetting your hair with warm water and then applying the hair conditioner to your hair.

4. Let it sit in for 15 to 30 minutes before you wash off.

Essential Oil Facial Toner

Ingredients

1 oz.fl., High Proof Vodka

8 drops Grapefruit Oil

2 1/2 oz.fl., Witch Hazel Hydrosol

4 drops Cypress Oil

4 ounce bottle

4 drops Tea Tree Oil

Instructions

1. In a clean and sterile glass bottle,

2. Combine vodka, grapefruit oil, witch hazel hydrosol, cypress oil and tea tree oil together.

3. Shake well to combine.

4. Shake thoroughly before use.

NOTE: Shaking thoroughly disperses the essential oils and prevents essential oil concentration.

5. Apply to your face after shaking properly with a cotton ball.

NOTE: Do not use drugstore bought witch hazel has it already contains alcohol.

Solid Sugar Cube Scrub Recipe

Sugar scrubs that are natural are known to always exfoliate and gently polish the skin, and they are far better compared to the abrasive and more synthetic variations available in the market. Their smells are out of this world and very natural.

Most natural sugar scrubs often separate over time, and this can be a nuisance to work with them; though they have so many great advantages. I have written this recipe to the correct the weaknesses found in most natural sugar cube scrubs. This sugar cube scrubs are easy to work with and are very attractive compared to scrubs that separate over time. They last very long when stored in the right way.

Ingredients

Makes: Thirty 1 inch square exfoliating sugar cubes.

11 net weight ounces Soap Base

2 cups White Sugar

4 oz.fl., Cold Pressed Vegetable Oil (use stable lipids like jojoba oil, watermelon seed Oil or fractionated coconut oil)

1/4 teaspoon Vitamin E oil)

1/4 oz.fl., (1 1/2 teaspoon) Essential Oil

Rectangular soap molds

Surgical gloves (needed while working)

Instructions

1. Melt soap base in a double boiler until it is melted completely.

NOTE: Don't overheat so that you dint ruin the soap lather.

2. In a mixing bowl, pour melted soap base.

3. Quickly toss in the Vitamin E oils and vegetable oils into the bowl and stir to combine.

NOTE: You need to be as quick as possible after instruction 1.

4. Toss sugar in and keep stirring.

TIP: Be fast when stirring and tossing in ingredients, because the mixture has tendencies of firming up pretty fast.

5. Knead soap base mixture with your gloved hands.

6. Measure in the essential oils and combine until the essential oil is well incorporated.

NOTE: If the mixture feels very thin, add more sugar until desired consistency is reached.

7. Scoop mixture into soap molds, making sure there are no air traps.

8. Keep aside to set for one hour.

NOTE: The rate at which mixture firms up is dependent on the quality and types of ingredients used. If the mixture appears too thing, refrigerate for a while.

9. Unmold the scrubs before the mixture sets completely; making it very easy to cut the cubes.

10. Cut into 1 inch cubes and allow to firm up for many hours at room temperature.

11. Don't use on skin areas with wounds, abrasions and cuts or if you have eczema. These scrubs can be used on the body and face, avoid the face.

12 Best used within 1 month and 1 ½ months.

Brush-On Cuticle Oil Recipe

During winter the weather becomes really tough on the cuticles and the surrounding skin. This recipe helps to keep the cuticles and the surrounding skin soft and winterproofed.

Ingredients

1/2 fluid oz. cranberry seed oil or any cold pressed carrier/vegetable oil that is rich in EFAs

5-8 drops tea tree or lavender essential oils

Instructions

1. Get a nail polish bottle or a small roller bottle or a small bottle with dropper tip,

2. Measure in carrier oil into the cleaned and sterile bottle.

3. Using a pipette or a dropper, measure in the essential oils into the bottle.

NOTE: sandalwood or patchouli essential oils can be a substitute for tea tree or lavender essential oil

4. Shake vigorously to incorporate essential oil well.

5. Shake before each application.

6. Brush nail polish bottle content onto your cuticles and the skin surrounding and massage it in.

NOTE: You can use as frequently as you desire.

7. Store well and don't use beyond 2 weeks after production.

Body Powder Recipe

This is an absorbent body powder that is free of talc.

Ingredients

30 drops Lavender Essential Oil or any other essential oil you like

4 oz. Body Powder Sifter Container

4 net weight oz. Arrowroot Powder

Instructions

1. In a large mixing bowl, measure in arrow root powder or non GMO (Genetically Modified Organism) cornstarch.

NOTE: Arrowroot is a little more expensive compared to the cornstarch, but it gives a silkier feel. For a skin that is oily, use 1/2 ounce white kaolin powder to substitute the cornstarch/arrowroot powder.

2. Toss in the essential oil and mix well to incorporate.

3. Transfer into a body powder sifter container.

4. Avoid the mucous membranes, the eyes, genitals, mouth and any other sensitive areas of the body.

Apply as you would a regular body powder.

NOTE: Adhere to all essential oil safety precautions when using any essential oil or blend. Always do a skin patch test for essential oils before usage, make sure the essential oils you are using are gentle to the skin.

Nourishing Lotion Recipe

Ingredients

8 oz.fl., unscented body or hand lotion

10 drops Patchouli essential oil

5 drops Carrot Seed essential oil

20 drops Sandalwood essential oil

Instructions

1. In a mixing bowl, measure in the unscented hand or body lotion.

2. Measure in patchouli oil, carrot seed oil, and sandal wood oil into the bowl.

3. Mix very well to incorporate essential oils into the lotion.

4. With a funnel, transfer bowl's content into a clean nd sterile glass bottle.

5. Apply as you would regular body and hand lotion.

TIP: Sandalwood oil, patchouli oil and carrot seed oil helps dry skin, Sandalwood oil and patchouli oils have a rich and lovely aroma when blended together, the carrot seed oil is great for the skin but has a little harsh scent compared to the other two.

NOTE: Adhere to all essential oil safety precautions when using any essential oil or blend. Always do a skin patch test for essential oils before usage, make sure the essential oils you are using are gentle to the skin.

Bath Salts Recipe

To fix the issue of essential oils not mixing with water, for this recipe we are going to use a solubilizer to minimize the risk of essential oils separating from water and coming in direct contact with our skin. We will be considering Polysorbate 20 or Solubol

Ingredients

3 cups salt (Epsom salt, Dead Sea Salt, Sea Salt, Himalayan Pink Salt)

1 tbsp Jojoba or any other carrier oil

15 drops favorite essential oil(s)

Solubol or Polysorbate 20 Solubilizer.

Instructions

1. Mix the essential oil and carrier oil together,

2. Measure in the solubilizer and mix well.

3. In another mixing bowl, add the salt or salts in.

4. Toss in essential oil mixture carefully into the bowl containing salts.

5. With a fork or a spoon, mix salt mixture thoroughly.

6. Get a salt tube, jar or container that covers well.

7. Transfer salts mixture into container and cover well.

NOTE: Salts stored in containers that do not cover well will lose their savor faster.

8. Set aside for a day, and shake well to incorporate essential oils well into the salt mixture.

9. In a running water bath tub, measure in 1/2 to 1 cup of the salts mixture into the tub, and mix thoroughly, to ensure thorough mixing before you enter the tub.

NOTE: Add bath salts just before you enter into the tub, to keep the essential oils from evaporating too soon. Make sure the salts dissolves well before entering into the tub, sitting or standing on large chunks of salts can be very painful.

NOTE 1: Any of the salts listed in this recipe can be used or a combination of these salts. Salts come in many different grain-sizes. Mixing two salts or several of them can make your salts a very pleasant sight to behold. Large grain sizes of salts are more appealing but they can be a little awkward and painful if you sit or step upon few undissolved pieces, and they take a long while before dissolving in the tub.

NOTE 2: Adhere to all essential oil safety precautions when using any essential oil or blend. Always do a skin patch test for essential oils before usage, make sure the essential oils you are using are gentle to the skin.

Bath Oil Recipe

Ingredients

2 oz.fl., Jojoba or any other carrier oil

Solubol or Polysorbate 20 Solubilizer

20 drops Lavender Essential Oil

Instructions

I. Combine carrier oil and essential oil together.

2. Measure in the solubilizer and mix well.

3. Transfer mixture into a clean and sterile glass bottle.

NOTE: This recipe may be increased.

4. Measure in approx. (7 to 8ml) 1/4 oz of bath oil into your bath water.

5. Mix very well before hopping into the tub, be sure essential oil have dispersed well in the water to avoid sensitization.

NOTE: Every few minutes wave your hands in the water to keep the bath oil mixture from settling in one spot.

Bath Bombs Recipe

This easy to make recipe is very pleasant and appealing when dropped into the tub. After the first and second time, it becomes second nature to make natural bath bombs. Making bath bombs would save you half of the store bought price and it would also help you to be sure that the ingredients are all natural.

Ingredients

1 cup Baking Soda

1/4 teaspoon Powdered Herbs or 1/8 teaspoon Pearlescent Mica {for color and appeal} (not compulsory)

1/2 cup Citric Acid

1/4 - 1/2 teaspoon Jojoba or any other stable carrier Oil

15 drops Essential Oil

Hydrosol or water

Surgical gloves

Instructions

1. Measure in baking soda, powdered herbs or pearlescent mica and citric acid into a large mixing bowl.

2. Stir thoroughly to free clumps.

3. Stir in the essential oil into the large bowl's content, drop by drop.

NOTE: The mixture might fix a little.

4. Gently add in vegetable or carrier oil as you mix the large bowl's contents with your hand.

5. Carefully measure in the hydrosol to the baking soda mixture using a spray bottle, as you keep blending with your hands.

NOTE: Measure in the water or hydrosol drop by drop, it doesn't take much liquid to dampen mixture to the amount needed to form bath bombs. So be careful not to over flood with liquids or moisten too much.

6. Press mixture into molds (you can use melon ballers, or try out soap, ice or candy molds of varying sizes and shapes).

7. Set molds on wax paper and set aside for 1 day to dry.

8. For a fizzy and aromatic bath, you should drop 1-2 bath bombs into your bath tub.

9. Store bath bombs in an well covered bag or container to retain their fizz.

NOTE: Store your citric acid well in a properly covered container to help retain its "fizzing" power.

10. Can stay up to 6 months if stored properly.

NOTE: If you are using strong essential oils such as geranium, adjust essential oil quantity.

Acne Aromatherapy Recipe

Ingredients

1 oz.fl., Jojoba or Fractionated Coconut Oil

5 drops Tea Tree Oil

6 drops Lavender Oil

1 drop Geranium Oil

Instructions

1. In a well cleaned amber glass bottle, measure in Jojoba or fractionated coconut oil.

2. Measure in tea tree oil, lavender oil and Geranium oil into the glass bottle.

NOTE: Undiluted essential oils shouldn't be stored in bottles with rubber tops. It is okay to store this recipe in a dropper top bottle, because it has been well diluted.

3. Gently mix the bottle's content by rolling the bottle for 1-2 minutes.

4. Avoid application of recipe to the lips, eyes, inside the ears and nostrils. Limit application of recipe to the face, back and neck in small amounts.

CHAPTER FIVE - ESSENTIAL OILS FOR EMOTIONS AND AROMATIC BLENDS

6 Aromatic Blend Options for Winter Blues Ease

The cold temperature, reduced activity, lack of greenery, snow covered world and gray skies can all accumulate and lead to what is known as the Winter Blues. This aromatic blend relieves the symptoms of winter blues by the use of uplifting essential oils for you and your household

NOTE: Remember and adhere to all essential oil safety precautions, when using and selecting oils. And do not use aromatherapy as a substitute for proper medical treatments.

Aromatic Blend Option 1

2 drops Grapefruit

3 drops Orange

Aromatic Blend Option 2

1 drop Ylang Ylang

4 drops Orange

Aromatic Blend Option 3

2 drops Ginger

3 drops Orange

Aromatic Blend Option 4

2 drops Cypress

3 drops Grapefruit

Aromatic Blend Option 5

2 drops Clary Sage

3 drops Bergamot

Aromatic Blend Option 6

1 drop Neroli

3 drops Bergamot

1 drop Jasmine

Instructions

Choose an option from one of the blend options listed above and use the method that best suites you from the instructions below.

For Bath Oils

1. Multiply any choice blend you have selected by 3 to make 15 drops of oils in total.

2. Combine 2 oz.fl., Jojoba oil or any other carrier oil and essential oil together.

3. Measure in solubol or Polysorbate 20 Solubilizer and mix well.

4. Transfer mixture into a clean and sterile glass bottle.

5. Measure in approx. (7 to 8ml) 1/4 oz of bath oil into your bath water.

6. Mix very well before hopping into the tub, be sure essential oil have dispersed well in the water to avoid sensitization.

NOTE: Every few minutes wave your hands in the water to keep the bath oil mixture from settling in one spot.

For Diffuser Blends

1. Multiply any choice blend you have selected by 4 to make 20 drops of oils in total.

2. Measure in essential oils into a bottle that is dark in color and mix thoroughly.

TIP: To mix essential oils in the bottle, roll bottle between your two hands.

3. Follow the instructions on the diffuser's manual and measure in the right amount from the blend created into the diffuser

For Bath Salts

1. Multiply any choice blend you have selected by 3 to make 15 drops of oils in total.

2. Mix the essential oils and 1 teaspoon of Jojoba or any other suitable carrier oil together,

3. Measure in the Solubol or Polysorbate 20 Solubilizer and mix well.

4. In another mixing bowl, add 3 cups salt (Epsom salt, Dead Sea Salt, Sea Salt, Himalayan Pink Salt).

5. Toss in essential oil mixture carefully into the bowl containing salts.

6. With a fork or a spoon, mix salt mixture thoroughly.

7. Get a salt tube, jar or container that covers well.

8. Transfer salts mixture into container and cover well.

NOTE: Salts stored in containers that do not cover well will lose their savor faster.

9. Set aside for a day, and shake well to incorporate essential oils well into the salt mixture.

10. In a running water bath tub, measure in 1/2 to 1 cup of the salts mixture into the tub, and mix thoroughly, to ensure thorough mixing before you enter the tub.

NOTE 1: Add bath salts just before you enter into the tub, to keep the essential oils from evaporating too soon. Make sure the salts dissolves well before entering into the tub, sitting or standing on large chunks of salts can be very painful.

NOTE 2: Any of the salts listed in this recipe can be used or a combination of these salts. Salts come in many different grain-sizes. Mixing two salts or several of them can make your salts a very pleasant sight to behold. Large grain sizes of salts are more appealing but they can be a little awkward and painful if you sit or step upon few undissolved pieces, and they take a long while before dissolving in the tub.

NOTE 3: Adhere to all essential oil safety precautions when using any essential oil or blend. Always do a skin patch test for essential oils before usage, make sure the essential oils you are using are gentle to the skin.

For Massage Oil

1. Multiply any choice blend you have selected by 2 to make 10 drops of oils in total.

2. Combine essential oils and sweet almond oil or any other suitable carrier oil together

3. Mix well.

4. Transfer essential oils mixture into a well covered dark glass jar/bottle/container.

5. Use ½ to 1 tsp during each massage.

17 Essential Oil Diffuser Recipes

Seventeen beautiful scented recipes designed for your olefactory pleasure that can be used with your essential oil diffuser.

Diffuser Blend Recipe 1

12 drops Patchouli

2 drops Linden Blossom

5 drops Vanilla

1 drop Neroli

Diffuser Blend Recipe 2

1 drop Jasmine

3 drops Sweet Orange

5 drops Lime

1 drop Cinnamon

Diffuser Blend Recipe 3

1 drop Jasmine

4 drops Bergamot

3 drops Sandalwood

2 drops Grapefruit

Diffuser Blend Recipe 4

4 drops Bergamot

2 drops Grapefruit

2 drops Lemon

2 drops Ylang Ylang

Diffuser Blend Recipe 5

10 drops Lime

2 drops Ylang Ylang

7 drops Bergamot

1 drop Rose

Diffuser Blend Recipe 6

4 drops Rosewood

1 drop Ylang Ylang

5 drops Lavender

Diffuser Blend Recipe 7

5 drops Spruce

2 drops Lavender

3 drops Cedar (Virginian)

Diffuser Blend Recipe 8

5 drops Rosemary

3 drops Lavender

1 drop Peppermint

1 drop Roman Chamomile

Diffuser Blend Recipe 9

5 drops Bergamot

1 drop Cypress

4 drops Lavender

Diffuser Blend Recipe 10

6 drops Bergamot

3 drops Spearmint

11 drops Lemon

Diffuser Blend Recipe 11

5 drops Spearmint

9 drops Sweet Orange

5 drops Lavender

Diffuser Blend Recipe 12

1 drop Jasmine

3 drops Patchouli

6 drops Sweet Orange

Diffuser Blend Recipe 13

5 drops Sandalwood

2 drops Lemon

1 drop Rose

2 drops Scotch pine

Diffuser Blend Recipe 14

4 drops Ylang Yalng

2 drops Bergamot

4 drops Clary Sage

Diffuser Blend Recipe 15

6 drops Juniper

1 drop Cinnamon

3 drops Sweet Orange

Diffuser Blend Recipe 16

7 drops Sweet Orange

1 drop Ylang Ylang

2 drops Vanilla

Diffuser Blend Recipe 17

9 drops Sandalwood

1 drop Neroli

Instructions:

Choose an option from one of the blend options listed above and use the method that best suites you from the instructions below.

1. Most blends are in 10 or 20 drops batches; select your choice blend,

2. Measure in essential oils into a bottle that is dark in color and mix thoroughly.

TIP: To mix essential oils in the bottle, roll bottle between your two hands.

3. Follow the instructions on the diffuser's manual and measure in the right amount from the blend created into the diffuser

NOTE: Get to know each essential oil's safety precaution and contraindication before use.

Absolutes and essential oils that are thick (vetivert, oakmoss, patchouli, benzoin, sandalwood) should be used carefully in nebulizing diffusers. Refer to your instructional manual for specific information.

4 Aromatic Blend Options for Stress Relief

Stress Relief Blend Option 1

2 drops Roman Chamomile Oil

1 drop Vetiver Oil

2 drops Lavender Oil

Stress Relief Blend Option 2

3 drops Clary Sage Oil

1 drop Lavender Oil

1 drop Lemon Oil

Stress Relief Blend Option 3

3 drops Grapefruit Oil

1 drop Ylang Ylang Oil

1 drop Jasmine Oil

Stress Relief Blend Option 4

3 drops Bergamot Oil

1 drop Frankincense Oil

1 drop Geranium Oil

Instructions

Choose an option from one of the blend options listed above and use the method that best suites you from the instructions below.

For Diffuser Blends

1. Multiply any choice blend you have selected by 4 to make 20 drops of oils in total.

2. Measure in essential oils into a bottle that is dark in color and mix thoroughly.

TIP: To mix essential oils in the bottle, roll bottle between your two hands.

3. Follow the instructions on the diffuser's manual and measure in the right amount from the blend created into the diffuser

For Bath Salts

1. Multiply any choice blend you have selected by 3 to make 15 drops of oils in total.

2. Mix the essential oils and 1 teaspoon of Jojoba or any other suitable carrier oil together,

3. Measure in the Solubol or Polysorbate 20 Solubilizer and mix well.

4. In another mixing bowl, add 3 cups salt (Epsom salt, Dead Sea Salt, Sea Salt, Himalayan Pink Salt).

5. Toss in essential oil mixture carefully into the bowl containing salts.

6. With a fork or a spoon, mix salt mixture thoroughly.

7. Get a salt tube, jar or container that covers well.

8. Transfer salts mixture into container and cover well.

NOTE: Salts stored in containers that do not cover well will lose their savor faster.

9. Set aside for a day, and shake well to incorporate essential oils well into the salt mixture.

10. In a running water bath tub, measure in ½ to 1 cup of the salts mixture into the tub, and mix thoroughly, to ensure thorough mixing before you enter the tub.

NOTE 1: Add bath salts just before you enter into the tub, to keep the essential oils from evaporating too soon. Make sure the salts dissolves well before entering into the tub, sitting or standing on large chunks of salts can be very painful.

NOTE 2: Any of the salts listed in this recipe can be used or a combination of these salts. Salts come in many different grain-sizes. Mixing two salts or several of them can make your salts a very pleasant sight to behold. Large grain sizes of salts are more appealing but they can be a little awkward and painful if you sit or step upon few undissolved pieces, and they take a long while before dissolving in the tub.

NOTE 3: Adhere to all essential oil safety precautions when using any essential oil or blend. Always do a skin patch test for essential oils before usage, make sure the essential oils you are using are gentle to the skin.

For Bath Oils

1. Multiply any choice blend you have selected by 3 to make 15 drops of oils in total.

2. Combine 2 oz.fl., Jojoba oil or any other carrier oil and essential oil together.

3. Measure in solubol or Polysorbate 20 Solubilizer and mix well.

4. Transfer mixture into a clean and sterile glass bottle.

5. Measure in approx. (7 to 8ml) 1/4 oz of bath oil into your bath water.

6. Mix very well before hopping into the tub, be sure essential oil have dispersed well in the water to avoid sensitization.

NOTE: Every few minutes wave your hands in the water to keep the bath oil mixture from settling in one spot.

For Massage Oil

1. Multiply any choice blend you have selected by 2 to make 10 drops of oils in total.

2. Combine essential oils and sweet almond oil or any other suitable carrier oil together

3. Mix well.

4. Transfer essential oils mixture into a well covered dark glass jar/bottle/container.

5. Use 1/2 to 1 tsp during each massage.

NOTE: Remember and adhere to all essential oil safety precautions, when using and selecting oils. And do not use aromatherapy as a substitute for proper medical treatments.

4 Aromatic Blend Options for Panic and Panic Attacks Relief

Panic and Panic Attacks Relief Blend Option 1

3 drops Frankincense

2 drops Helichrysum

Panic and Panic Attacks Relief Blend Option 2

4 drops Lavender

1 drop Neroli

Panic and Panic Attacks Relief Blend Option 3

4 drops Lavender

1 drop Rose

Panic and Panic Attacks Relief Blend Option 4

4 drops Frankincense

1 drops Rose

Instructions

Choose an option from one of the blend options listed above and use the method that best suites you from the instructions below.

For Diffuser Blends

1. Multiply any choice blend you have selected by 4 to make 20 drops of oils in total.

2. Measure in essential oils into a bottle that is dark in color and mix thoroughly.

TIP: To mix essential oils in the bottle, roll bottle between your two hands.

3. Follow the instructions on the diffuser's manual and measure in the right amount from the blend created into the diffuser

For Bath Salts

1. Multiply any choice blend you have selected by 3 to make 15 drops of oils in total.

2. Mix the essential oils and 1 teaspoon of Jojoba or any other suitable carrier oil together,

3. Measure in the Solubol or Polysorbate 20 Solubilizer and mix well.

4. In another mixing bowl, add 3 cups salt (Epsom salt, Dead Sea Salt, Sea Salt, Himalayan Pink Salt).

5. Toss in essential oil mixture carefully into the bowl containing salts.

6. With a fork or a spoon, mix salt mixture thoroughly.

7. Get a salt tube, jar or container that covers well.

8. Transfer salts mixture into container and cover well.

NOTE: Salts stored in containers that do not cover well will lose their savor faster.

9. Set aside for a day, and shake well to incorporate essential oils well into the salt mixture.

10. In a running water bath tub, measure in 1/2 to 1 cup of the salts mixture into the tub, and mix thoroughly, to ensure thorough mixing before you enter the tub.

NOTE 1: Add bath salts just before you enter into the tub, to keep the essential oils from evaporating too soon. Make sure the salts dissolves well before entering into the tub, sitting or standing on large chunks of salts can be very painful.

NOTE 2: Any of the salts listed in this recipe can be used or a combination of these salts. Salts come in many different grain-sizes. Mixing two salts or several of them can make your salts a very pleasant sight to behold. Large grain sizes of salts are more appealing but they can be a little awkward and painful if you sit or step upon few undissolved pieces, and they take a long while before dissolving in the tub.

NOTE 3: Adhere to all essential oil safety precautions when using any essential oil or blend. Always do a skin patch test for essential oils before usage, make sure the essential oils you are using are gentle to the skin.

For Bath Oils

1. Multiply any choice blend you have selected by 3 to make 15 drops of oils in total.

2. Combine 2 oz.fl., Jojoba oil or any other carrier oil and essential oil together.

3. Measure in solubol or Polysorbate 20 Solubilizer and mix well.

4. Transfer mixture into a clean and sterile glass bottle.

5. Measure in approx. (7 to 8ml) 1/4 oz of bath oil into your bath water.

6. Mix very well before hopping into the tub, be sure essential oil have dispersed well in the water to avoid sensitization.

NOTE: Every few minutes wave your hands in the water to keep the bath oil mixture from settling in one spot.

For Massage Oil

1. Multiply any choice blend you have selected by 2 to make 10 drops of oils in total.

2. Combine essential oils and sweet almond oil or any other suitable carrier oil together

3. Mix well.

4. Transfer essential oils mixture into a well covered dark glass jar/bottle/container.

5. Use 1/2 to 1 tsp during each massage.

NOTE: Remember and adhere to all essential oil safety precautions, when using and selecting oils. And do not use aromatherapy as a substitute for proper medical treatments.

5 Aromatic Blend Options for Memory and Concentration Enhancement

Some essential oils are famed for their ability to enhance concentration and memory, essential oils like rosemary oils. Cypress essential oil, lemon essential oil and peppermint essential oil can be very helpful in staying alert and focused.

Memory and Concentration Enhancement Blend Option 1

2 drops Lemon

3 drops Rosemary

Memory and Concentration Enhancement Blend Option 2

1 drop Basil

2 drops Cypress

2 drops Rosemary

Memory and Concentration Enhancement Blend Option 3

1 drops Peppermint

4 drops Cypress

Memory and Concentration Enhancement Blend Option 4

3 drops Lemon

2 drops Peppermint

Memory and Concentration Enhancement Blend Option 5

2 drops Hyssop

3 drops Lemon

Instructions

Choose an option from one of the blend options listed above and use the method that best suites you from the instructions below.

For Diffuser Blends

1. Multiply any choice blend you have selected by 4 to make 20 drops of oils in total.

2. Measure in essential oils into a bottle that is dark in color and mix thoroughly.

TIP: To mix essential oils in the bottle, roll bottle between your two hands.

3. Follow the instructions on the diffuser's manual and measure in the right amount from the blend created into the diffuser

For Bath Salts

1. Multiply any choice blend you have selected by 3 to make 15 drops of oils in total.

2. Mix the essential oils and 1 teaspoon of Jojoba or any other suitable carrier oil together,

3. Measure in the Solubol or Polysorbate 20 Solubilizer and mix well.

4. In another mixing bowl, add 3 cups salt (Epsom salt, Dead Sea Salt, Sea Salt, Himalayan Pink Salt).

5. Toss in essential oil mixture carefully into the bowl containing salts.

6. With a fork or a spoon, mix salt mixture thoroughly.

7. Get a salt tube, jar or container that covers well.

8. Transfer salts mixture into container and cover well.

NOTE: Salts stored in containers that do not cover well will lose their savor faster.

9. Set aside for a day, and shake well to incorporate essential oils well into the salt mixture.

10. In a running water bath tub, measure in 1/2 to 1 cup of the salts mixture into the tub, and mix thoroughly, to ensure thorough mixing before you enter the tub.

NOTE 1: Add bath salts just before you enter into the tub, to keep the essential oils from evaporating too soon. Make sure the salts dissolves well before entering into the tub, sitting or standing on large chunks of salts can be very painful.

NOTE 2: Any of the salts listed in this recipe can be used or a combination of these salts. Salts come in many different grain-sizes. Mixing two salts or several of them can make your salts a very pleasant sight to behold. Large grain sizes of salts are more appealing but they can be a little awkward and painful if you sit or step upon few undissolved pieces, and they take a long while before dissolving in the tub.

NOTE 3: Adhere to all essential oil safety precautions when using any essential oil or blend. Always do a skin patch test for essential oils before usage, make sure the essential oils you are using are gentle to the skin.

For Bath Oils

1. Multiply any choice blend you have selected by 3 to make 15 drops of oils in total.

2. Combine 2 oz.fl., Jojoba oil or any other carrier oil and essential oil together.

3. Measure in solubol or Polysorbate 20 Solubilizer and mix well.

4. Transfer mixture into a clean and sterile glass bottle.

5. Measure in approx. (7 to 8ml) 1/4 oz of bath oil into your bath water.

6. Mix very well before hopping into the tub, be sure essential oil have dispersed well in the water to avoid sensitization.

NOTE: Every few minutes wave your hands in the water to keep the bath oil mixture from settling in one spot.

For Massage Oil

1. Multiply any choice blend you have selected by 2 to make 10 drops of oils in total.

2. Combine essential oils and sweet almond oil or any other suitable carrier oil together

3. Mix well.

4. Transfer essential oils mixture into a well covered dark glass jar/bottle/container.

5. Use 1/2 to 1 tsp during each massage.

NOTE: Remember and adhere to all essential oil safety precautions, when using and selecting oils. And do not use aromatherapy as a substitute for proper medical treatments.

4 Aromatic Blend Options for Loneliness Relief

Loneliness Relief Blend Option 1

2 drops Frankincense

1 drop Rose

2 drops Bergamot

Loneliness Relief Blend Option 2

2 drops Roman Chamomile

3 drops Bergamot

Loneliness Relief Blend Option 3

3 drops Clary Sage

2 drops Bergamot

Loneliness Relief Blend Option 4

3 drops Clary Sage

2 drops Frankincense

Instructions

Choose an option from one of the blend options listed above and use the method that best suites you from the instructions below.

For Diffuser Blends

1. Multiply any choice blend you have selected by 4 to make 20 drops of oils in total.

2. Measure in essential oils into a bottle that is dark in color and mix thoroughly.

TIP: To mix essential oils in the bottle, roll bottle between your two hands.

3. Follow the instructions on the diffuser's manual and measure in the right amount from the blend created into the diffuser

For Bath Salts

1. Multiply any choice blend you have selected by 3 to make 15 drops of oils in total.

2. Mix the essential oils and 1 teaspoon of Jojoba or any other suitable carrier oil together,

3. Measure in the Solubol or Polysorbate 20 Solubilizer and mix well.

4. In another mixing bowl, add 3 cups salt (Epsom salt, Dead Sea Salt, Sea Salt, Himalayan Pink Salt).

5. Toss in essential oil mixture carefully into the bowl containing salts.

6. With a fork or a spoon, mix salt mixture thoroughly.

7. Get a salt tube, jar or container that covers well.

8. Transfer salts mixture into container and cover well.

NOTE: Salts stored in containers that do not cover well will lose their savor faster.

9. Set aside for a day, and shake well to incorporate essential oils well into the salt mixture.

10. In a running water bath tub, measure in 1/2 to 1 cup of the salts mixture into the tub, and mix thoroughly, to ensure thorough mixing before you enter the tub.

NOTE 1: Add bath salts just before you enter into the tub, to keep the essential oils from evaporating too soon. Make sure the salts dissolves well before entering into the tub, sitting or standing on large chunks of salts can be very painful.

NOTE 2: Any of the salts listed in this recipe can be used or a combination of these salts. Salts come in many different grain-sizes. Mixing two salts or several of them can make your salts a very pleasant sight to behold. Large grain sizes of salts are more appealing but they can be a little awkward and painful if you sit or step upon few undissolved pieces, and they take a long while before dissolving in the tub.

NOTE 3: Adhere to all essential oil safety precautions when using any essential oil or blend. Always do a skin patch test for essential oils before usage, make sure the essential oils you are using are gentle to the skin.

For Bath Oils

1. Multiply any choice blend you have selected by 3 to make 15 drops of oils in total.

2. Combine 2 oz.fl., Jojoba oil or any other carrier oil and essential oil together.

3. Measure in solubol or Polysorbate 20 Solubilizer and mix well.

4. Transfer mixture into a clean and sterile glass bottle.

5. Measure in approx. (7 to 8ml) 1/4 oz of bath oil into your bath water.

6. Mix very well before hopping into the tub, be sure essential oil have dispersed well in the water to avoid sensitization.

NOTE: Every few minutes wave your hands in the water to keep the bath oil mixture from settling in one spot.

For Massage Oil

1. Multiply any choice blend you have selected by 2 to make 10 drops of oils in total.

2. Combine essential oils and sweet almond oil or any other suitable carrier oil together

3. Mix well.

4. Transfer essential oils mixture into a well covered dark glass jar/bottle/container.

5. Use 1/2 to 1 tsp during each massage.

NOTE: Remember and adhere to all essential oil safety precautions, when using and selecting oils. And do not use aromatherapy as a substitute for proper medical treatments.

5 Aromatic Blend Options for Irritability Reduction

Irritability Reduction Blend Option 1

2 drops Lavender

3 drops Mandarin

Irritability Reduction Blend Option 2

4 drops Sandalwood

1 drop Neroli

Irritability Reduction Blend Option 3

2 drops Lavender

2 drops Roman Chamomile

1 drop Neroli

Irritability Reduction Blend Option 4

2 drops Mandarin

3 drops Roman Chamomile

Irritability Reduction Blend Option 5

3 drops Sandalwood

2 drops Mandarin

Instructions

Choose an option from one of the blend options listed above and use the method that best suites you from the instructions below.

For Diffuser Blends

1. Multiply any choice blend you have selected by 4 to make 20 drops of oils in total.

2. Measure in essential oils into a bottle that is dark in color and mix thoroughly.

TIP: To mix essential oils in the bottle, roll bottle between your two hands.

3. Follow the instructions on the diffuser's manual and measure in the right amount from the blend created into the diffuser

For Bath Salts

1. Multiply any choice blend you have selected by 3 to make 15 drops of oils in total.

2. Mix the essential oils and 1 teaspoon of Jojoba or any other suitable carrier oil together,

3. Measure in the Solubol or Polysorbate 20 Solubilizer and mix well.

4. In another mixing bowl, add 3 cups salt (Epsom salt, Dead Sea Salt, Sea Salt, Himalayan Pink Salt).

5. Toss in essential oil mixture carefully into the bowl containing salts.

6. With a fork or a spoon, mix salt mixture thoroughly.

7. Get a salt tube, jar or container that covers well.

8. Transfer salts mixture into container and cover well.

NOTE: Salts stored in containers that do not cover well will lose their savor faster.

9. Set aside for a day, and shake well to incorporate essential oils well into the salt mixture.

10. In a running water bath tub, measure in 1/2 to 1 cup of the salts mixture into the tub, and mix thoroughly, to ensure thorough mixing before you enter the tub.

NOTE 1: Add bath salts just before you enter into the tub, to keep the essential oils from evaporating too soon. Make sure the salts dissolves well before entering into the tub, sitting or standing on large chunks of salts can be very painful.

NOTE 2: Any of the salts listed in this recipe can be used or a combination of these salts. Salts come in many different grain-sizes. Mixing two salts or several of them can make your salts a very pleasant sight to behold. Large grain sizes of salts are more appealing but they can be a little awkward and painful if you sit or step upon few undissolved pieces, and they take a long while before dissolving in the tub.

NOTE 3: Adhere to all essential oil safety precautions when using any essential oil or blend. Always do a skin patch test for essential oils before usage, make sure the essential oils you are using are gentle to the skin.

For Bath Oils

1. Multiply any choice blend you have selected by 3 to make 15 drops of oils in total.

2. Combine 2 oz.fl., Jojoba oil or any other carrier oil and essential oil together.

3. Measure in solubol or Polysorbate 20 Solubilizer and mix well.

4. Transfer mixture into a clean and sterile glass bottle.

5. Measure in approx. (7 to 8ml) 1/4 oz of bath oil into your bath water.

6. Mix very well before hopping into the tub, be sure essential oil have dispersed well in the water to avoid sensitization.

NOTE: Every few minutes wave your hands in the water to keep the bath oil mixture from settling in one spot.

For Massage Oil

1. Multiply any choice blend you have selected by 2 to make 10 drops of oils in total.

2. Combine essential oils and sweet almond oil or any other suitable carrier oil together.

3. Mix well.

4. Transfer essential oils mixture into a well covered dark glass jar/bottle/container.

5. Use 1/2 to 1 tsp during each massage.

NOTE: Remember and adhere to all essential oil safety precautions, when using and selecting oils. And do not use aromatherapy as a substitute for proper medical treatments.

Aromatic Blend for Insomnia and Trouble Sleeping Relief

The root cause of insomnia cannot be cured by Aromatherapy. This recipe guarantees relaxing and calming essential oils that can potentially extend your sleeping time. Help you sleep faster and wake up at the time of your desire.

For chronic sleep disorders refer to health professionals for diagnosis and proper treatment.

Ingredients

5 drops Bergamot Essential Oil

10 drops Roman Chamomile Essential Oil

5 drops Clary Sage Essential Oil

Instructions

1. Get a clean and sterile bottle that is dark in color.

2. Measure in bergamot, roman chamomile, and clary sage essential oils into the bottle.

3. Mix essential oils in the bottle, roll the bottle between your two hands.

4. Add 1 to 2 drops to a tissue paper.

5. Keep tissue paper inside the pillow before you sleep.

NOTE: Do not allow the essential oils come in direct contact with your skin or face.

For Diffuser Blend

If you prefer to make a diffuser blend that you enjoy during the hour before bedtime, make a blend with a ratio of 2 drops Roman Chamomile to 1 drop Clary Sage to 1 drop Bergamot and add to your diffuser.

Lavender Essential Oil can also help provide relaxation and drowsiness, but using more than 1-2 drops can have the opposite effect.

For a diffuser blend, should be enjoyed one hour before your intended sleeping time.

1. Measure in essential oils into a bottle that is dark in color and mix thoroughly.

TIP: To mix essential oils in the bottle, roll bottle between your two hands.

2. Follow the instructions on the diffuser's manual and measure in the right amount from the blend created into the diffuser.

4 Aromatic Blend Options for Insecurity Relief

Insecurity Relief Blend Option 1

3 drops Bergamot

1 drop Vetiver

1 drop Jasmine

Insecurity Relief Blend Option 2

1 drop Jasmine

4 drops Sandalwood

Insecurity Relief Blend Option 3

2 drops Cedarwood

1 drop Frankincense

2 drops Bergamot

Insecurity Relief Blend Option 4

2 drops Frankincense

3 drops Sandalwood

Instructions

Choose an option from one of the blend options listed above and use the method that best suites you from the instructions below.

For Diffuser Blends

1. Multiply any choice blend you have selected by 4 to make 20 drops of oils in total.

2. Measure in essential oils into a bottle that is dark in color and mix thoroughly.

TIP: To mix essential oils in the bottle, roll bottle between your two hands.

3. Follow the instructions on the diffuser's manual and measure in the right amount from the blend created into the diffuser

For Bath Salts

1. Multiply any choice blend you have selected by 3 to make 15 drops of oils in total.

2. Mix the essential oils and 1 teaspoon of Jojoba or any other suitable carrier oil together,

3. Measure in the Solubol or Polysorbate 20 Solubilizer and mix well.

4. In another mixing bowl, add 3 cups salt (Epsom salt, Dead Sea Salt, Sea Salt, Himalayan Pink Salt).

5. Toss in essential oil mixture carefully into the bowl containing salts.

6. With a fork or a spoon, mix salt mixture thoroughly.

7. Get a salt tube, jar or container that covers well.

8. Transfer salts mixture into container and cover well.

NOTE: Salts stored in containers that do not cover well will lose their savor faster.

9. Set aside for a day, and shake well to incorporate essential oils well into the salt mixture.

10. In a running water bath tub, measure in 1/2 to 1 cup of the salts mixture into the tub, and mix thoroughly, to ensure thorough mixing before you enter the tub.

NOTE 1: Add bath salts just before you enter into the tub, to keep the essential oils from evaporating too soon. Make sure the salts dissolves well before entering into the tub, sitting or standing on large chunks of salts can be very painful.

NOTE 2: Any of the salts listed in this recipe can be used or a combination of these salts. Salts come in many different grain-sizes.

Mixing two salts or several of them can make your salts a very pleasant sight to behold. Large grain sizes of salts are more appealing but they can be a little awkward and painful if you sit or step upon few undissolved pieces, and they take a long while before dissolving in the tub.

NOTE 3: Adhere to all essential oil safety precautions when using any essential oil or blend. Always do a skin patch test for essential oils before usage, make sure the essential oils you are using are gentle to the skin.

For Bath Oils

1. Multiply any choice blend you have selected by 3 to make 15 drops of oils in total.

2. Combine 2 oz.fl., Jojoba oil or any other carrier oil and essential oil together.

3. Measure in solubol or Polysorbate 20 Solubilizer and mix well.

4. Transfer mixture into a clean and sterile glass bottle.

5. Measure in approx. (7 to 8ml) 1/4 oz of bath oil into your bath water.

6. Mix very well before hopping into the tub, be sure essential oil have dispersed well in the water to avoid sensitization.

NOTE: Every few minutes wave your hands in the water to keep the bath oil mixture from settling in one spot.

For Massage Oil

1. Multiply any choice blend you have selected by 2 to make 10 drops of oils in total.

2. Combine essential oils and sweet almond oil or any other suitable carrier oil together

3. Mix well.

4. Transfer essential oils mixture into a well covered dark glass jar/bottle/container.

5. Use 1/2 to 1 tsp during each massage.

NOTE: Remember and adhere to all essential oil safety precautions, when using and selecting oils. And do not use aromatherapy as a substitute for proper medical treatments.

4 Aromatic Blend Options for Happiness Enhancement

These recipes enhance peace, joy and happiness.

Happiness Enhancement Blend Option 1

3 drops Bergamot

1 drop Grapefruit

1 drop Ylang Ylang

Happiness Enhancement Blend Option 2

1 drop Geranium

2 drops Orange

2 drops Frankincense

Happiness Enhancement Blend Option 3

2 drops Sandalwood

2 drops Bergamot

1 drop Rose

Happiness Enhancement Blend Option 4

2 drops Orange or Lemon or Bergamot

1 drop Rose or Ylang Ylang or Neroli

2 drops Grapefruit

Instructions

Choose an option from one of the blend options listed above and use the method that best suites you from the instructions below.

For Diffuser Blends

1. Multiply any choice blend you have selected by 4 to make 20 drops of oils in total.

2. Measure in essential oils into a bottle that is dark in color and mix thoroughly.

TIP: To mix essential oils in the bottle, roll bottle between your two hands.

3. Follow the instructions on the diffuser's manual and measure in the right amount from the blend created into the diffuser

For Bath Salts

1. Multiply any choice blend you have selected by 3 to make 15 drops of oils in total.

2. Mix the essential oils and 1 teaspoon of Jojoba or any other suitable carrier oil together,

3. Measure in the Solubol or Polysorbate 20 Solubilizer and mix well.

4. In another mixing bowl, add 3 cups salt (Epsom salt, Dead Sea Salt, Sea Salt, Himalayan Pink Salt).

5. Toss in essential oil mixture carefully into the bowl containing salts.

6. With a fork or a spoon, mix salt mixture thoroughly.

7. Get a salt tube, jar or container that covers well.

8. Transfer salts mixture into container and cover well.

NOTE: Salts stored in containers that do not cover well will lose their savor faster.

9. Set aside for a day, and shake well to incorporate essential oils well into the salt mixture.

10. In a running water bath tub, measure in 1/2 to 1 cup of the salts mixture into the tub, and mix thoroughly, to ensure thorough mixing before you enter the tub.

NOTE 1: Add bath salts just before you enter into the tub, to keep the essential oils from evaporating too soon. Make sure the salts dissolves well before entering into the tub, sitting or standing on large chunks of salts can be very painful.

NOTE 2: Any of the salts listed in this recipe can be used or a combination of these salts. Salts come in many different grain-sizes. Mixing two salts or several of them can make your salts a very pleasant sight to behold. Large grain sizes of salts are more appealing but they can be a little awkward and painful if you sit or step upon few undissolved pieces, and they take a long while before dissolving in the tub.

NOTE 3: Adhere to all essential oil safety precautions when using any essential oil or blend. Always do a skin patch test for essential oils before usage, make sure the essential oils you are using are gentle to the skin.

For Bath Oils

1. Multiply any choice blend you have selected by 3 to make 15 drops of oils in total.

2. Combine 2 oz.fl., Jojoba oil or any other carrier oil and essential oil together.

3. Measure in solubol or Polysorbate 20 Solubilizer and mix well.

4. Transfer mixture into a clean and sterile glass bottle.

5. Measure in approx. (7 to 8ml) 1/4 oz of bath oil into your bath water.

6. Mix very well before hopping into the tub, be sure essential oil have dispersed well in the water to avoid sensitization.

NOTE: Every few minutes wave your hands in the water to keep the bath oil mixture from settling in one spot.

For Massage Oil

1. Multiply any choice blend you have selected by 2 to make 10 drops of oils in total.

2. Combine essential oils and sweet almond oil or any other suitable carrier oil together.

3. Mix well.

4. Transfer essential oils mixture into a well covered dark glass jar/bottle/container.

5. Use 1/2 to 1 tsp during each massage.

NOTE: Remember and adhere to all essential oil safety precautions, when using and selecting oils. And do not use aromatherapy as a substitute for proper medical treatments.

4 Aromatic Blend Options for Grief Help

Rose oil is generally known to be of great help during moments of grief.

Grief Help Blend Option 1

3 drops Sandalwood

2 drops Rose

Grief Help Blend Option 2

1 drop Neroli

3 drops Sandalwood

1 drop Rose

Grief Help Blend Option 3

3 drops Cypress

2 drops Rose

Grief Help Blend Option 4

1 drop Rose

1 drop Cypress

1 drop Helichrysum

2 drops Frankincense

Instructions

Choose an option from one of the blend options listed above and use the method that best suites you from the instructions below.

For Diffuser Blends

1. Multiply any choice blend you have selected by 4 to make 20 drops of oils in total.

2. Measure in essential oils into a bottle that is dark in color and mix thoroughly.

TIP: To mix essential oils in the bottle, roll bottle between your two hands.

3. Follow the instructions on the diffuser's manual and measure in the right amount from the blend created into the diffuser

For Bath Salts

1. Multiply any choice blend you have selected by 3 to make 15 drops of oils in total.

2. Mix the essential oils and 1 teaspoon of Jojoba or any other suitable carrier oil together,

3. Measure in the Solubol or Polysorbate 20 Solubilizer and mix well.

4. In another mixing bowl, add 3 cups salt (Epsom salt, Dead Sea Salt, Sea Salt, Himalayan Pink Salt).

5. Toss in essential oil mixture carefully into the bowl containing salts.

6. With a fork or a spoon, mix salt mixture thoroughly.

7. Get a salt tube, jar or container that covers well.

8. Transfer salts mixture into container and cover well.

NOTE: Salts stored in containers that do not cover well will lose their savor faster.

9. Set aside for a day, and shake well to incorporate essential oils well into the salt mixture.

10. In a running water bath tub, measure in 1/2 to 1 cup of the salts mixture into the tub, and mix thoroughly, to ensure thorough mixing before you enter the tub.

NOTE 1: Add bath salts just before you enter into the tub, to keep the essential oils from evaporating too soon. Make sure the salts dissolves well before entering into the tub, sitting or standing on large chunks of salts can be very painful.

NOTE 2: Any of the salts listed in this recipe can be used or a combination of these salts. Salts come in many different grain-sizes. Mixing two salts or several of them can make your salts a very pleasant sight to behold. Large grain sizes of salts are more appealing but they can be a little awkward and painful if you sit or step upon few undissolved pieces, and they take a long while before dissolving in the tub.

NOTE 3: Adhere to all essential oil safety precautions when using any essential oil or blend. Always do a skin patch test for essential oils before usage, make sure the essential oils you are using are gentle to the skin.

For Bath Oils

1. Multiply any choice blend you have selected by 3 to make 15 drops of oils in total.

2. Combine 2 oz.fl., Jojoba oil or any other carrier oil and essential oil together.

3. Measure in solubol or Polysorbate 20 Solubilizer and mix well.

4. Transfer mixture into a clean and sterile glass bottle.

5. Measure in approx. (7 to 8ml) 1/4 oz of bath oil into your bath water.

6. Mix very well before hopping into the tub, be sure essential oil have dispersed well in the water to avoid sensitization.

NOTE: Every few minutes wave your hands in the water to keep the bath oil mixture from settling in one spot.

For Massage Oil

1. Multiply any choice blend you have selected by 2 to make 10 drops of oils in total.

2. Combine essential oils and sweet almond oil or any other suitable carrier oil together

3. Mix well.

4. Transfer essential oils mixture into a well covered dark glass jar/bottle/container.

5. Use 1/2 to 1 tsp during each massage.

NOTE: Remember and adhere to all essential oil safety precautions, when using and selecting oils. And do not use aromatherapy as a substitute for proper medical treatments.

4 Aromatic Blend Options for Easing Fear

Fear Easing Blend Option 1

Also works at moments when you need energy.

2 drops Bergamot

3 drops Grapefruit

Fear Easing Blend Option 2

2 drops Orange

3 drops Sandalwood

Fear Easing Blend Option 3

Also works at moments when you need calm and to relax.

2 drops Clary Sage

1 drop Vetiver

2 drops Roman Chamomile

Fear Easing Blend Option 4

2 drops Jasmine or 2 drops Neroli

1 drop Clary Sage

2 drops Frankincense

Instructions

Choose an option from one of the blend options listed above and use the method that best suites you from the instructions below.

For Diffuser Blends

1. Multiply any choice blend you have selected by 4 to make 20 drops of oils in total.

2. Measure in essential oils into a bottle that is dark in color and mix thoroughly.

TIP: To mix essential oils in the bottle, roll bottle between your two hands.

3. Follow the instructions on the diffuser's manual and measure in the right amount from the blend created into the diffuser

For Bath Salts

1. Multiply any choice blend you have selected by 3 to make 15 drops of oils in total.

2. Mix the essential oils and 1 teaspoon of Jojoba or any other suitable carrier oil together,

3. Measure in the Solubol or Polysorbate 20 Solubilizer and mix well.

4. In another mixing bowl, add 3 cups salt (Epsom salt, Dead Sea Salt, Sea Salt, Himalayan Pink Salt).

5. Toss in essential oil mixture carefully into the bowl containing salts.

6. With a fork or a spoon, mix salt mixture thoroughly.

7. Get a salt tube, jar or container that covers well.

8. Transfer salts mixture into container and cover well.

NOTE: Salts stored in containers that do not cover well will lose their savor faster.

9. Set aside for a day, and shake well to incorporate essential oils well into the salt mixture.

10. In a running water bath tub, measure in 1/2 to 1 cup of the salts mixture into the tub, and mix thoroughly, to ensure thorough mixing before you enter the tub.

NOTE 1: Add bath salts just before you enter into the tub, to keep the essential oils from evaporating too soon. Make sure the salts dissolves well before entering into the tub, sitting or standing on large chunks of salts can be very painful.

NOTE 2: Any of the salts listed in this recipe can be used or a combination of these salts. Salts come in many different grain-sizes. Mixing two salts or several of them can make your salts a very pleasant sight to behold. Large grain sizes of salts are more appealing but they can be a little awkward and painful if you sit or step upon few undissolved pieces, and they take a long while before dissolving in the tub.

NOTE 3: Adhere to all essential oil safety precautions when using any essential oil or blend. Always do a skin patch test for essential oils before usage, make sure the essential oils you are using are gentle to the skin.

For Bath Oils

1. Multiply any choice blend you have selected by 3 to make 15 drops of oils in total.

2. Combine 2 oz.fl., Jojoba oil or any other carrier oil and essential oil together.

3. Measure in solubol or Polysorbate 20 Solubilizer and mix well.

4. Transfer mixture into a clean and sterile glass bottle.

5. Measure in approx. (7 to 8ml) 1/4 oz of bath oil into your bath water.

6. Mix very well before hopping into the tub, be sure essential oil have dispersed well in the water to avoid sensitization.

NOTE: Every few minutes wave your hands in the water to keep the bath oil mixture from settling in one spot.

For Massage Oil

1. Multiply any choice blend you have selected by 2 to make 10 drops of oils in total.

2. Combine essential oils and sweet almond oil or any other suitable carrier oil together

3. Mix well.

4. Transfer essential oils mixture into a well covered dark glass jar/bottle/container.

5. Use 1/2 to 1 tsp during each massage.

NOTE: Remember and adhere to all essential oil safety precautions, when using and selecting oils. And do not use aromatherapy as a substitute for proper medical treatments

4 Aromatic Blend Options For Energy and Staying Alert

Energy and Staying Alert Blend Option 1

2 drops Basil

2 drops Grapefruit

1 drop Cypress

Energy and Staying Alert Blend Option 2

3 drops Bergamot

2 drops Rosemary

Energy and Staying Alert Blend Option 3

2 drops Ginger

3 drops Grapefruit

Energy and Staying Alert Blend Option 4

1 drop Frankincense

2 drops Peppermint

2 drops Lemon

Instructions

Choose an option from one of the blend options listed above and use the method that best suites you from the instructions below.

For Diffuser Blends

1. Multiply any choice blend you have selected by 4 to make 20 drops of oils in total.

2. Measure in essential oils into a bottle that is dark in color and mix thoroughly.

TIP: To mix essential oils in the bottle, roll bottle between your two hands.

3. Follow the instructions on the diffuser's manual and measure in the right amount from the blend created into the diffuser

For Bath Salts

1. Multiply any choice blend you have selected by 3 to make 15 drops of oils in total.

2. Mix the essential oils and 1 teaspoon of Jojoba or any other suitable carrier oil together,

3. Measure in the Solubol or Polysorbate 20 Solubilizer and mix well.

4. In another mixing bowl, add 3 cups salt (Epsom salt, Dead Sea Salt, Sea Salt, Himalayan Pink Salt).

5. Toss in essential oil mixture carefully into the bowl containing salts.

6. With a fork or a spoon, mix salt mixture thoroughly.

7. Get a salt tube, jar or container that covers well.

8. Transfer salts mixture into container and cover well.

NOTE: Salts stored in containers that do not cover well will lose their savor faster.

9. Set aside for a day, and shake well to incorporate essential oils well into the salt mixture.

10. In a running water bath tub, measure in 1/2 to 1 cup of the salts mixture into the tub, and mix thoroughly, to ensure thorough mixing before you enter the tub.

NOTE 1: Add bath salts just before you enter into the tub, to keep the essential oils from evaporating too soon. Make sure the salts dissolves well before entering into the tub, sitting or standing on large chunks of salts can be very painful.

NOTE 2: Any of the salts listed in this recipe can be used or a combination of these salts. Salts come in many different grain-sizes. Mixing two salts or several of them can make your salts a very pleasant sight to behold. Large grain sizes of salts are more appealing but they can be a little awkward and painful if you sit or step upon few undissolved pieces, and they take a long while before dissolving in the tub.

NOTE 3: Adhere to all essential oil safety precautions when using any essential oil or blend. Always do a skin patch test for essential oils before usage, make sure the essential oils you are using are gentle to the skin.

For Bath Oils

1. Multiply any choice blend you have selected by 3 to make 15 drops of oils in total.

2. Combine 2 oz.fl., Jojoba oil or any other carrier oil and essential oil together.

3. Measure in solubol or Polysorbate 20 Solubilizer and mix well.

4. Transfer mixture into a clean and sterile glass bottle.

5. Measure in approx. (7 to 8ml) 1/4 oz of bath oil into your bath water.

6. Mix very well before hopping into the tub, be sure essential oil have dispersed well in the water to avoid sensitization.

NOTE: Every few minutes wave your hands in the water to keep the bath oil mixture from settling in one spot.

For Massage Oil

1. Multiply any choice blend you have selected by 2 to make 10 drops of oils in total.

2. Combine essential oils and sweet almond oil or any other suitable carrier oil together

3. Mix well.

4. Transfer essential oils mixture into a well covered dark glass jar/bottle/container.

5. Use 1/2 to 1 tsp during each massage.

NOTE: Remember and adhere to all essential oil safety precautions, when using and selecting oils. And do not use aromatherapy as a substitute for proper medical treatments.

4 Aromatic blend Options for Depression relief

Depression Relief Blend Option 1

1 drop Rose

1 drop Orange

3 drops Sandalwood

Depression Relief Blend Option 2

1 drop Lavender

3 drops Grapefruit

1 drop Ylang Ylang

Depression Relief Blend Option 3

2 drops Clary Sage

3 drops Bergamot

Depression Relief Blend Option 4

2 drops Frankincense

2 drops Jasmine or Neroli

1 drop Lemon

Instructions

Choose an option from one of the blend options listed above and use the method that best suites you from the instructions below.

For Diffuser Blends

1. Multiply any choice blend you have selected by 4 to make 20 drops of oils in total.

2. Measure in essential oils into a bottle that is dark in color and mix thoroughly.

TIP: To mix essential oils in the bottle, roll bottle between your two hands.

3. Follow the instructions on the diffuser's manual and measure in the right amount from the blend created into the diffuser

For Bath Salts

1. Multiply any choice blend you have selected by 3 to make 15 drops of oils in total.

2. Mix the essential oils and 1 teaspoon of Jojoba or any other suitable carrier oil together,

3. Measure in the Solubol or Polysorbate 20 Solubilizer and mix well.

4. In another mixing bowl, add 3 cups salt (Epsom salt, Dead Sea Salt, Sea Salt, Himalayan Pink Salt).

5. Toss in essential oil mixture carefully into the bowl containing salts.

6. With a fork or a spoon, mix salt mixture thoroughly.

7. Get a salt tube, jar or container that covers well.

8. Transfer salts mixture into container and cover well.

NOTE: Salts stored in containers that do not cover well will lose their savor faster.

9. Set aside for a day, and shake well to incorporate essential oils well into the salt mixture.

10. In a running water bath tub, measure in 1/2 to 1 cup of the salts mixture into the tub, and mix thoroughly, to ensure thorough mixing before you enter the tub.

NOTE 1: Add bath salts just before you enter into the tub, to keep the essential oils from evaporating too soon. Make sure the salts dissolves well before entering into the tub, sitting or standing on large chunks of salts can be very painful.

NOTE 2: Any of the salts listed in this recipe can be used or a combination of these salts. Salts come in many different grain-sizes. Mixing two salts or several of them can make your salts a very pleasant sight to behold. Large grain sizes of salts are more appealing but they can be a little awkward and painful if you sit or step upon few undissolved pieces, and they take a long while before dissolving in the tub.

NOTE 3: Adhere to all essential oil safety precautions when using any essential oil or blend. Always do a skin patch test for essential oils before usage, make sure the essential oils you are using are gentle to the skin.

For Bath Oils

1. Multiply any choice blend you have selected by 3 to make 15 drops of oils in total.

2. Combine 2 oz.fl., Jojoba oil or any other carrier oil and essential oil together.

3. Measure in solubol or Polysorbate 20 Solubilizer and mix well.

4. Transfer mixture into a clean and sterile glass bottle.

5. Measure in approx. (7 to 8ml) 1/4 oz of bath oil into your bath water.

6. Mix very well before hopping into the tub, be sure essential oil have dispersed well in the water to avoid sensitization.

NOTE: Every few minutes wave your hands in the water to keep the bath oil mixture from settling in one spot.

For Massage Oil

1. Multiply any choice blend you have selected by 2 to make 10 drops of oils in total.

2. Combine essential oils and sweet almond oil or any other suitable carrier oil together

3. Mix well.

4. Transfer essential oils mixture into a well covered dark glass jar/bottle/container.

5. Use 1/2 to 1 tsp during each massage.

NOTE: Remember and adhere to all essential oil safety precautions, when using and selecting oils. And do not use aromatherapy as a substitute for proper medical treatments.

Aromatic Blend for Calm and Relaxing

Ingredients

1 Oz.fl., Sweet almond oil or any other suitable carrier oil

5 drops Lavender

7 drops Roman Chamomile

Instructions

1. Combine lavender, Roman chamomile and sweet almond oil together.

2. Measure in essential oils into a well covered bottle that is dark in color and mix thoroughly.

TIP: To mix essential oils in the bottle, roll bottle between your two hands.

3. Apply as a body or massage oil. You can apply as feet massage oil also.

NOTE: Do not drive after use, because Lavender and Roman chamomile are natural sedatives.

For Diffuser Blends

If you prefer to use a diffuser instead, make a diffuser blend with lavender and Roman Chamomile having ratios 1:2. For Examples 2 drops of lavender to 4 drops of Roman chamomile.

1. Measure in essential oils into a bottle that is dark in color and mix thoroughly.

TIP: To mix essential oils in the bottle, roll bottle between your two hands.

2. Follow the instructions on the diffuser's manual and measure in the right amount from the blend created into the diffuser.

4 Aromatic Blend Options for Boosting Confidence

Confidence Booster Blend Option 1

3 drops Bergamot

2 drops Bay Laurel

Confidence Booster Blend Option 2

1 drop Jasmine

4 drops Bergamot

Confidence Booster Blend Option 3

2 drops Rosemary

3 drops Orange

Confidence Booster Blend Option 4

2 drops Cypress

3 drops Grapefruit

Instructions

Choose an option from one of the blend options listed above and use the method that best suites you from the instructions below.

For Diffuser Blends

1. Multiply any choice blend you have selected by 4 to make 20 drops of oils in total.

2. Measure in essential oils into a bottle that is dark in color and mix thoroughly.

TIP: To mix essential oils in the bottle, roll bottle between your two hands.

3. Follow the instructions on the diffuser's manual and measure in the right amount from the blend created into the diffuser

For Bath Salts

1. Multiply any choice blend you have selected by 3 to make 15 drops of oils in total.

2. Mix the essential oils and 1 teaspoon of Jojoba or any other suitable carrier oil together,

3. Measure in the Solubol or Polysorbate 20 Solubilizer and mix well.

4. In another mixing bowl, add 3 cups salt (Epsom salt, Dead Sea Salt, Sea Salt, Himalayan Pink Salt).

5. Toss in essential oil mixture carefully into the bowl containing salts.

6. With a fork or a spoon, mix salt mixture thoroughly.

7. Get a salt tube, jar or container that covers well.

8. Transfer salts mixture into container and cover well.

NOTE: Salts stored in containers that do not cover well will lose their savor faster.

9. Set aside for a day, and shake well to incorporate essential oils well into the salt mixture.

10. In a running water bath tub, measure in 1/2 to 1 cup of the salts mixture into the tub, and mix thoroughly, to ensure thorough mixing before you enter the tub.

NOTE 1: Add bath salts just before you enter into the tub, to keep the essential oils from evaporating too soon. Make sure the salts dissolves well before entering into the tub, sitting or standing on large chunks of salts can be very painful.

NOTE 2: Any of the salts listed in this recipe can be used or a combination of these salts. Salts come in many different grain-sizes. Mixing two salts or several of them can make your salts a very pleasant sight to behold. Large grain sizes of salts are more appealing but they can be a little awkward and painful if you sit or step upon few undissolved pieces, and they take a long while before dissolving in the tub.

NOTE 3: Adhere to all essential oil safety precautions when using any essential oil or blend. Always do a skin patch test for essential oils before usage, make sure the essential oils you are using are gentle to the skin.

For Bath Oils

1. Multiply any choice blend you have selected by 3 to make 15 drops of oils in total.

2. Combine 2 oz.fl., Jojoba oil or any other carrier oil and essential oil together.

3. Measure in solubol or Polysorbate 20 Solubilizer and mix well.

4. Transfer mixture into a clean and sterile glass bottle.

5. Measure in approx. (7 to 8ml) 1/4 oz of bath oil into your bath water.

6. Mix very well before hopping into the tub, be sure essential oil have dispersed well in the water to avoid sensitization.

NOTE: Every few minutes wave your hands in the water to keep the bath oil mixture from settling in one spot.

For Massage Oil

1. Multiply any choice blend you have selected by 2 to make 10 drops of oils in total.

2. Combine essential oils and sweet almond oil or any other suitable carrier oil together

3. Mix well.

4. Transfer essential oils mixture into a well covered dark glass jar/bottle/container.

5. Use 1/2 to 1 tsp during each massage.

NOTE: Remember and adhere to all essential oil safety precautions, when using and selecting oils. And do not use aromatherapy as a substitute for proper medical treatments.

Essential Oil Diffuser Recipe for Giving Thanks, Celebrating and Expressing Gratitude

1. Grapefruit

This essential oil gives deliciously fragrance that uplifts.

2. Bergamot

Loved by everyone for its sweet and soft fragrance that uplifts. Can be used as a part of any blend meant for celebration or to enhance joy as primary oil.

3. Ylang Ylang

This essential oil has floral and exotic characteristics which can be really strong: so I advice to use little amounts. Jasmine is a good substitute also.

4. Frankincense

Frankincense is an essential oil that has spicy and earthy base notes to help give great fragrances. To celebrate gratitude and faith, this essential oil is the answer.

5. Cypress

This essential oil has fresh, slightly woody and herbal fragrances, and it is widely known as an essential oil that enhances energy. This is a great essential oil option during times of change.

6. Ginger

This essential oil is warming and an uplifting spicy oil that helps complement the sweetness of ylang ylang essential oil and citrus essential oil.

Ingredients

20 drops Bergamot

10 drops Cypress

10 drops Grapefruit

5 drops Ylang Ylang

10 Drops Frankincese

2 drops Ginger

Instructions

For Diffuser Blends

1. Measure in Bergamot, cypress, grapefruit, ylang ylang, frankincense and ginger essential oils into a bottle that is dark in color and mix thoroughly.

TIP: To mix essential oils in the bottle, roll bottle between your two hands.

2. Follow the instructions on the diffuser's manual and measure in the right amount from the blend created into the diffuser

NOTE: You can experiment carefully and discover newer blends.

4 Aromatic Blend Option for Anxiety Relief

Anxiety Relief Blend Option 1

2 drops Bergamot

1 drop Frankincense

2 drops Clary Sage

Anxiety Relief Blend Option 2

2 drops Clary Sage

3 drops Lavender

Anxiety Relief Blend Option 3

2 drops Bergamot

3 drops Sandalwood

Anxiety Relief Blend Option 4

1 drop Rose

2 drops Mandarin

1 drop Lavender

1 drop Vetiver

Instructions

Choose an option from one of the blend options listed above and use the method that best suites you from the instructions below.

For Diffuser Blends

1. Multiply any choice blend you have selected by 4 to make 20 drops of oils in total.

2. Measure in essential oils into a bottle that is dark in color and mix thoroughly.

TIP: To mix essential oils in the bottle, roll bottle between your two hands.

3. Follow the instructions on the diffuser's manual and measure in the right amount from the blend created into the diffuser.

For Bath Salts

1. Multiply any choice blend you have selected by 3 to make 15 drops of oils in total.

2. Mix the essential oils and 1 teaspoon of Jojoba or any other suitable carrier oil together,

3. Measure in the Solubol or Polysorbate 20 Solubilizer and mix well.

4. In another mixing bowl, add 3 cups salt (Epsom salt, Dead Sea Salt, Sea Salt, Himalayan Pink Salt).

5. Toss in essential oil mixture carefully into the bowl containing salts.

6. With a fork or a spoon, mix salt mixture thoroughly.

7. Get a salt tube, jar or container that covers well.

8. Transfer salts mixture into container and cover well.

NOTE: Salts stored in containers that do not cover well will lose their savor faster.

9. Set aside for a day, and shake well to incorporate essential oils well into the salt mixture.

10. In a running water bath tub, measure in 1/2 to 1 cup of the salts mixture into the tub, and mix thoroughly, to ensure thorough mixing before you enter the tub.

NOTE 1: Add bath salts just before you enter into the tub, to keep the essential oils from evaporating too soon. Make sure the salts dissolves well before entering into the tub, sitting or standing on large chunks of salts can be very painful.

NOTE 2: Any of the salts listed in this recipe can be used or a combination of these salts. Salts come in many different grain-sizes. Mixing two salts or several of them can make your salts a very pleasant sight to behold. Large grain sizes of salts are more appealing but they can be a little awkward and painful if you sit or step upon few undissolved pieces, and they take a long while before dissolving in the tub.

NOTE 3: Adhere to all essential oil safety precautions when using any essential oil or blend. Always do a skin patch test for essential oils before usage, make sure the essential oils you are using are gentle to the skin.

For Bath Oils

1. Multiply any choice blend you have selected by 3 to make 15 drops of oils in total.

2. Combine 2 oz.fl., Jojoba oil or any other carrier oil and essential oil together.

3. Measure in solubol or Polysorbate 20 Solubilizer and mix well.

4. Transfer mixture into a clean and sterile glass bottle.

5. Measure in approx. (7 to 8ml) 1/4 oz of bath oil into your bath water.

6. Mix very well before hopping into the tub, be sure essential oil have dispersed well in the water to avoid sensitization.

NOTE: Every few minutes wave your hands in the water to keep the bath oil mixture from settling in one spot.

For Massage Oil

1. Multiply any choice blend you have selected by 2 to make 10 drops of oils in total.

2. Combine essential oils and sweet almond oil or any other suitable carrier oil together

3. Mix well.

4. Transfer essential oils mixture into a well covered dark glass jar/bottle/container.

5. Use 1/2 to 1 tsp during each massage.

NOTE: Remember and adhere to all essential oil safety precautions, when using and selecting oils. And do not use aromatherapy as a substitute for proper medical treatments.

4 Aromatic Blend Options for Anger Management

Anger Management Blend Option 1

1 drop Rose

1 drop Vetiver

3 drops Orange

Anger Management Blend Option 2

1 drop Roman Chamomile

2 drops Orange

2 drops Bergamot

Anger Management Blend Option 3

3 drops Bergamot

1 drop Jasmine

1 drop Ylang Ylang

Anger Management Blend Option 4

2 drops Patchouli

3 drops Orange

Instructions

Choose an option from one of the blend options listed above and use the method that best suites you from the instructions below.

For Diffuser Blends

1. Multiply any choice blend you have selected by 4 to make 20 drops of oils in total.

2. Measure in essential oils into a bottle that is dark in color and mix thoroughly.

TIP: To mix essential oils in the bottle, roll bottle between your two hands.

3. Follow the instructions on the diffuser's manual and measure in the right amount from the blend created into the diffuser

For Bath Salts

1. Multiply any choice blend you have selected by 3 to make 15 drops of oils in total.

2. Mix the essential oils and 1 teaspoon of Jojoba or any other suitable carrier oil together,

3. Measure in the Solubol or Polysorbate 20 Solubilizer and mix well.

4. In another mixing bowl, add 3 cups salt (Epsom salt, Dead Sea Salt, Sea Salt, Himalayan Pink Salt).

5. Toss in essential oil mixture carefully into the bowl containing salts.

6. With a fork or a spoon, mix salt mixture thoroughly.

7. Get a salt tube, jar or container that covers well.

8. Transfer salts mixture into container and cover well.

NOTE: Salts stored in containers that do not cover well will lose their savor faster.

9. Set aside for a day, and shake well to incorporate essential oils well into the salt mixture.

10. In a running water bath tub, measure in 1/2 to 1 cup of the salts mixture into the tub, and mix thoroughly, to ensure thorough mixing before you enter the tub.

NOTE 1: Add bath salts just before you enter into the tub, to keep the essential oils from evaporating too soon. Make sure the salts dissolves well before entering into the tub, sitting or standing on large chunks of salts can be very painful.

NOTE 2: Any of the salts listed in this recipe can be used or a combination of these salts. Salts come in many different grain-sizes. Mixing two salts or several of them can make your salts a very pleasant sight to behold. Large grain sizes of salts are more appealing but they can be a little awkward and painful if you sit or step upon few undissolved pieces, and they take a long while before dissolving in the tub.

NOTE 3: Adhere to all essential oil safety precautions when using any essential oil or blend. Always do a skin patch test for essential oils before usage, make sure the essential oils you are using are gentle to the skin.

For Bath Oils

1. Multiply any choice blend you have selected by 3 to make 15 drops of oils in total.

2. Combine 2 oz.fl., Jojoba oil or any other carrier oil and essential oil together.

3. Measure in solubol or Polysorbate 20 Solubilizer and mix well.

4. Transfer mixture into a clean and sterile glass bottle.

5. Measure in approx. (7 to 8ml) 1/4 oz of bath oil into your bath water.

6. Mix very well before hopping into the tub, be sure essential oil have dispersed well in the water to avoid sensitization.

NOTE: Every few minutes wave your hands in the water to keep the bath oil mixture from settling in one spot.

For Massage Oil

1. Multiply any choice blend you have selected by 2 to make 10 drops of oils in total.

2. Combine essential oils and sweet almond oil or any other suitable carrier oil together

3. Mix well.

4. Transfer essential oils mixture into a well covered dark glass jar/bottle/container.

5. Use 1/2 to 1 tsp during each massage.

NOTE: Remember and adhere to all essential oil safety precautions, when using and selecting oils. And do not use aromatherapy as a substitute for proper medical treatments.

CHAPTER SIX - ESSENTIAL OILS FOR FIRST AID AND HEALTH

Aromatherapy Minor Scrapes and Cuts Recipe

Ingredients

Cotton Ball

5-6 drops Lavender Essential Oil

1 oz. Witch Hazel Hydrosol

Glass bottle

Instructions

1. Combine Lavender essential oil and hydrosol into a clean and sterile glass bottle.

2. Shake well by rolling the bottle between both hands.

3. To apply, soak cottonball with a little amount of the bottle's content

4. Since lavender brings calm, you can smell the cotton ball to allow the soothing scent calm your nerves, then apply to the minor cut or scrape.

5. If you deem it necessary, apply a band aid.

Minor Scrapes and Cuts Balm Recipe

Antibiotic ointments generally contain petroleum jelly. And Petroleum jelly is derived from the production of petroleum, it is manmade and it is known to clog pores. Instead of the regular petroleum jelly as an ingredient, we are using vegetable oils and beeswax. This makes it a strong antibiotic ointment alternative.

Ingredients

3 oz.fl., Sweet Almond Oil/Jojoba oil or any other suitable vegetable carrier oil

40 drops Lavender Oil

1 net weight oz. Beeswax, grated

4 oz Jar, (with a wide mouth)

40 drops Tea Tree Oil

Instructions

1. In a double boiler at low heat, place the grated beeswax in.

NOTE: Make sure you remember that it is difficult to remove beeswax from pans.

2. Heat sweet almond oil or Jojoba oil or any other carrier oil you have chosen, slowly and gently.

3. In a small bowl, transfer the carrier oil after heating.

4. Measure in the melted beeswax into the carrier oil bowl and then stir to combine.

5. Measure in the tea tree essential oil and lavender essential oil into the bowl and stir to incorporate the essential oils.

6. Transfer whole mixture into the jar with a wide mouth.

7. Set aside to cool for approx. 5 minutes before covering.

8 Apply only after the ointment has cooled sufficiently.

9. Clean minor scrapes and cuts and apply balm in small amounts and if you feel the need, you can bandage cuts.

Aromatherapy Blend for Congestion

Ingredients

30 drops Eucalyptus Essential Oil

4 drops Peppermint Essential Oil

26 drops Ravensara Essential Oil

Aromatherapy Inhaler or Cotton Ball

Instructions

1. Combine eucalyptus, peppermint, ravensara together.

2. Transfer into a clean and sterile bottle that is dark.

TIP: A bottle with a built in dropper insert would be a great choice.

3. Drop 2 to 3 drops on a cotton ball and draw or sniff in through your nostril. If you are using a new aromatherapy inhaler, dip the insert into the essential oil blend and return into the tube as you lock the lid in place. Inhale aromatherapy inhaler and take a long drag in through your nostril.

Massage Oil Recipe

Ingredients

1 oz.fl., Sweet almond oil or any other suitable carrier oil

10-12 drops of (complimenting) essential oils.

Stress Blend Option

6 drops Clary Sage

3 drops Lavender

2 drops Lemon

Restful Blend (Promoting Sleep) Option

5 drops Lavender

5 drops Roman Chamomile

Aphrodisiac Blend Option

2 drops Jasmine

8 drops Sandalwood

Sore Muscle Blend Option

2 drops Ginger

4 drops Peppermint

1 drops Black Pepper

5 drops Eucalyptus

Instructions

1. Combine essential oils and sweet almond oil or any other suitable carrier oil together

2. Mix well.

3. Transfer oils mixture into a well covered dark glass jar/bottle/container.

4. Use 1/2 to 1 tsp during each massage.

Aromatherapy for Menstrual Cramps Recipe

Cramps can be a nightmare of sorts for many women like me every time their period comes around. It can be really uncomfortable and painful, and can disrupt many other scheduled plans and activities. This recipe with a soothing massage is a fast relief combination that can help reduce the pains and discomforts gotten from menstrual cramps.

Ingredients

1 oz.fl. Jojoba

4 drops Cypress Essential Oil

5 drops Peppermint Essential Oil

3 drops Lavender Essential Oil

Instructions

1. Combine cypress, peppermint, lavender and Jojoba oils together

2. Mix well.

3. Transfer oils mixture into a well covered dark glass jar/bottle/container.

4. Apply a little amount to the abdominal area and massage.

Aromatherapy Blend for Bruises

Ingredients

8 drops Helichrysum Essential Oil

1 oz.fl., Sweet Almond or Jojoba Oil

Instructions

1. Combine Helichrysum into sweet almond or Jojoba oil

2. Mix well.

3. Transfer oils mixture into a well covered dark glass jar/bottle/container.

4. Apply a little amount to bruises once or twice daily.

NOTE: Other substitutes for helichrysum essential oil includes Roman chamomile, Yarrow and German Chamomile. They are all good anti-inflammatories and can be used together or as substitutes.

END

Thank you for reading my book. If you enjoyed it, won't you please take a moment to look at my other titles?

Thanks!

Carla Whites